I0476684

# Water for Wood

## Caregiver Relationship Compatibility based on the elements of Feng Shui

-a personal journey to compatible care relationships

Janet Ng

Janet Ng

## Dedication

*This book is dedicated to my mother, whose relationship with caregivers inspired the writing of this book.*

# Contents

# Introduction

My elderly mother has gone through more than 200 in-home caregivers over the past eighteen months due, in part, to incompatibility. She is sometimes referred to as a *special client*, because of her unpredictable mood swings. Some caregivers barely make it through the door before she orders them out of her home. Others walk out voluntarily after ten minutes of verbal abuse. Still others get along well with her, and stay for a very long time. The ones who choose to stay leave only due to spousal job transfers or career advancement, and not because of incompatibility. These caregivers truly love her, and she loves them – and yet, to me, they do not seem much different than the ones who leave under duress.

I began to wonder: what was the special ingredient - the common ground - that ignited a good connection? If I could figure it out, perhaps things would go better for her, as well as for me. She can intuit a bad match as soon as she looks at a potential caregiver. I do not have that sixth sense of knowing who will get along with her - but magically, she does.

Several years ago, I practiced Feng shui. I maintained a small website to assist people with furniture placement for improved health, wealth, relationships, and harmony; and provided relationship advice, based on compatibility between personal Feng shui elements. I received excellent feedback, and it was a lot of fun; but after a few years, my life became too busy to provide personal advice, so I gave it up. I did not think too much about the topic until my mother's constant parade of failed caregiver relationships brought the idea back to mind several months ago.

Mom is not the easiest client to work with. She's mercurial, demanding, and sometimes a little unkind to her caregivers due to the changes brought on by aging and cognitive decline. I initially thought she was the problem; then I noticed she got along very well with some of her caregivers – and wondered why? It was not necessarily about how good or bad a caregiver was, as I had seen her reject caregivers who seemed excellent, while she embraced others I would never have chosen for myself.

What is it that attracts her to some, and angers her with others? In her defense, there have been some who were total psychopaths - but I am referring to scenarios where two very nice people stand side by side: one of whom she is instantly taken by, while she glares at the other with a look of contempt I do not understand. There is either instant fondness or aversion; and if I debate with her, and convince her to give a rejected candidate a chance, it always ends in failure. The instinct she has about caregivers is directly related to the energy between them, which is either comfortable and familiar, or a negative vibration that makes her feel unsafe – a perception that comes from her gut, and it never fails.

I began to ask new applicants for their birth dates and calculated their Feng shui elements. What I discovered not only amazed me, but started to weigh heavily on future hiring decisions. My mother got along well with caregivers whose elements were harmonious with hers; while those with mismatched elements quickly walked off the job, or were terminated due to relational conflict.

My own metal element is not compatible with her wood element with me as the caregiver. Metal naturally controls wood, either constructively or destructively, and after a few weeks of trying to live in and care for her, I gave up the struggle of trying to get her to take medicine, eat healthy food, and wear oxygen – life supports she needed. We always got along well as mother and daughter, but apparently not in a situation where I provided her direct care. I became easily frustrated when I tried to get her to do the right things for her health - when what she really needed was care, not control.

She still uses caregivers, some from a team we hire privately, and others sent by an agency. I am able to find suitable matches for her private team, but have little control over who the agency sends. The turnover rate for the agency care givers has been outrageous, while very low for our private team, and usually due to a great match moving away, going back to school, or advancing her career.

What is considered *compatible* to my element is not the same for my mother; and when I mistakenly hire to suit my tastes, rather than her elemental needs, the relationship routinely fails. Therefore I no longer suggest that she hire caregivers not compatible with her element.

The combination of my metal element as a caregiver to my mother's wood element does not make a practical care relation, as mentioned above. The reason relates directly to nature. Wood represents trees and plants, while metal represents items such as silver, gold, pruning shears, or an axe. You might imagine how we get along when she is not cooperating with her care. I become impatient, and instinctively pull out my shears to *try* and prune her defiance for healthy living into submission.

Metal people simply do not have patience for contrary wood people - yet cropping of the person's branches is not conducive to the preservation of mental or emotional health of an elderly person already struggling to maintain dignity. I am not a bad person, yet have little to no business caring directly for a wood person who refuses to wear needed oxygen, or take medications. It is not in my makeup. Case closed. What I am good at is managing her affairs, which includes her caregivers, while leaving the direct care to those whose elements work best with hers.

**Ruthie** was one of the best caregivers Mom ever had, and worked with her for over a year. She is no longer with Mom because she got a promotion in her main job that left no time to be a caregiver.

Mom was filled with instant peace when Ruthie came on shift. They had a natural bond that was absent with most caregivers – yet easily understood in relation to their element combination.

Ruthie was born of water, which nurtured Mom's wood element. Watching them together via video camera was like witnessing gentle rain refresh a withering willow. Mom came to life when Ruthie was there, sometimes they stayed awake all night talking or watching movies. I did not worry when Ruthie was on shift, and slept all night sans loud phone calls from my mother about a caregiver she demanded I "get rid of." I was distressed when Ruthie announced she could not come anymore, having become accustomed to peaceful nights of sleep.

**Salena** is another caregiver who still works on our private team, after a year, and gets along well with Mom most of the time - yet their relationship is different than with Ruthie. Salena is earth, and actually gets along better with my metal element than with Mom's wood, as earth nurtures metal, yet is controlled by wood. She helps me a great deal by making doctor appointments, and a lot of other time-consuming tasks; however she is sometimes over-taxed emotionally by Mom's rapid mood swings.

Wood represents what grows from the earth – trees, plants, and flowers. A relationship between wood and earth is like that of a potted plant, with Mom being the plant, and Salena being the soil that feeds the plant. It is a perfect setup until the plant sucks all of the nutrients from the soil, leaving earth completely drained of what the plant continues to need to survive. The plant draws harder, and the soil becomes depleted.

Most gardeners would change the soil at this point to continue providing the plant with sufficient nutrition to thrive. What we have in Salena, however, is like Miracle-Grow potting mix because she manages to recharge herself, along with encouragement from me. I see it from time to time - the drain on Salena, as Mom's care demands sometimes outweigh Salena's reservoir of emotional stamina. That is when my metal jumps in, calls Mom, and talks her into easing up on Salena, while sprinkling words of praise over Salena's soil. It always works, and Salena gets an extra boost of energy in the process.

Earth does not know how to say "No" to wood because earth is like the mother to wood. Mom somehow intuits this, as she once asked Salena to be her new mother. Sometimes Mom gets confused, and thinks I am her mother. She was angry with me one day because I insisted she wear her oxygen, so decided to replace me with Salena.

Salena can nearly always be found by Mom's side, during her shift, catering to her needs or wants. She gets tired, and I have given her full permission to nap while Mom naps, allowing her to recharge for when Mom is awake and needing her constant attention.

**Sandy** was another awesome earth caregiver who found creative ways to care for Mom without becoming emotionally exhausted. She quit working with Mom three times, due to the strain, coming back every time because she really loved her; yet Mom's sometimes disturbing pull on Sandy's diminishing resources was strong, and she became easily sapped, and quit a fourth time. She returned after a few months, having finally found a way to nurture Mom, and recharge her own reserves. Sandy  is a harpist, and on occasion brought her portable harp to play for Mom, which soothed  Mom's soul, and refreshed her own. They were great together, but Sandy had to leave because she and her husband moved across the country to be closer to their children.

**Rita** was an earth caregiver who initially got along famously with Mom, but became unable to replace what Mom's wood element finally drained from her. Things got ugly as Rita's earth became completely sterile, which left her stressed out and bitter. As gardeners do, we had to replace the  potting soil via a different caregiver.

Mom lights up when **Tene** comes on shift. Tene is wood, like Mom, and the two of them seem more like friends – Tene, the peaceful willow, and Mom as the overgrown crabapple tree. Tene seems to have a natural understanding of Mom's moods, and instinctively gentles her to do what she should do, like wearing her oxygen. At first, Tene was afraid to coax Mom to wear the oxygen cannula. Mom yelled "No!" and Tene withdrew. I encouraged Tene to at least try. Tene finally understood the connection between their wood energies, and there was not another night without oxygen. She finally got the hang of gentling her into submission.

I have to say it was quite amusing watching the camera the first time Tene attempted to convince Mom to put her oxygen back on, without giving up. Picture the "Horse Whisperer" putting a bridal on a wild horse for the first time; nostrils flared, snorting, stamping hooves on the ground in threatening gesture. That depicts what Tene faced with Mom.

Tene slowly picked up the oxygen tube, and quietly backed away six paces from my mother's fury.

"Mrs. Smith," Tene said.

"What?!?! my mother said.

Mom's voice was sharp and loud, eyes narrowed, aimed directly at Tene, hoping to frighten her into retreat. Tene stood quietly, and continued to face my mother, seemingly unscathed by her venom. She waited a few seconds, then raised her hands slightly, and held the tubing in front of her in my mother's direction - eyes locked on Mom. First one step, then another, as she slowly moved toward my mother. Her hands extended ready to bridle that horse. As she took her final step, and reached toward Mom's nose to gently place the tubing, Mom reared back, throwing her hands up, and said,

"No!! Get that away from me!"

Tene stepped back again, waited, then repeated her determined journey to my mother's nostrils. Three times she tried, and was blasted away as many; but she did not give up. Tene took a slow, deep breath, and moved forward one more time, slowly pushing the tube in Mom's direction. Mom sat quietly as Tene gently placed the tube to her nose. No words were at first spoken, and then my mother looked up at Tene and quietly said,

"Thank you."

Tene said, "You're welcome, Mrs. Smith."

From that night forward, Tene has had no trouble helping my mother with her oxygen. The interaction between them was wood to wood, tree to tree, one branch bending to the other's touch, acceptance of the willow's wisp from a crabby tree. They have become kindred spirits in a world of inner torment that claws at my mother like a cat tied inside of a gunny sack.

**Jakeesha** was a caregiver my mother thoroughly enjoyed, but there was role reversal where Mom began taking care of the caregiver. Jakeesha took slight advantage, and attempted to drive a wedge between Mom and myself, while she tried to cozy my mother up to her own family members. She shared stories of woe which elicited sympathy, a hoped for response of offered cash beyond her normal pay. Of course I stopped the notion before it went further, which made Jakeesha all the more determined to influence Mom to spurn me. Jakeesha's element was fire, and she also *was* fired.

Fire gets along very well with wood, and becomes nurtured by the good smack of wood crackling beneath its flames. Mom's deceased husband was fire, and it was an agreeable arrangement in that Mom nurtured and cared for him. However, Jakeesha was supposed to care for Mom, and not the reverse. While the relationship between fire and wood is good, it is not necessarily the best match when the caregiver is fire.

**Veronica** was hired because she seemed like a suitable caregiver from my perspective. Mom did not like her at all, which I failed to understand. I talked with Mom until she reluctantly allowed me to hire her. Veronica's metal element was realized only after she accepted the job offer. My desire to hire her was apparently due to the good energy between she and I since we were both metal; yet mistakenly paired her metal with my wood mother, which was a regretted move.

Metal controls wood - and sometimes destructively. I coached Veronica about the elements, and that she would need to remain alert to any tendency to be bossy, irritable, or controlling with Mom. She tried, at first, to restrain her metal-to-wood tendencies, but as days went by, she gradually lost patience with Mom, and became verbally assaultive, more with each passing day - until finally she threatened and cussed, and frequently dropped the f-bomb to attempt control.

After repeated talks with Veronica, I terminated her for lack of acceptable caregiver behavior, coupled with concern that physical aggression might be soon to follow her unsuccessful verbal power attempts.

I vowed never again to hire another metal caregiver after Mom's experience with Veronica and myself as caregivers because both proved unsuccessful. Several more metal caregivers were interviewed, without at first realizing their element; but not hired, as the negative energy during employment discussions became apparent as Mom closed her eyes to avoid contact. I was no longer surprised by this type of negative reaction from Mom; but rather saw it as an indication of a bad potential match. Each metal applicant was nice and polite, but Mom was able to sense impending doom, even though not obvious to me. Mom is not aware of element philosophy, yet is almost magically able to sense incompatibility as soon as she looks a person in the eye.

I shared the element theory with the caregiver agency, as they supplied about a third of Mom's caregivers. They showed interest because of the constant staff renewal rate they experienced with Mom, and asked for the formula to calculate the elements. They hoped to have an easier time sending caregivers who might work well with her - especially after unwittingly sending metal caregivers, and spending a lot of time and grief clearing up messes caused by the metal-to-wood interaction. The agency and I are working together where possible to provide suitable caregiver matches, and though the process is not perfected, it is improving.

A caregiver's element is only half the equation, with the remainder being the general mental health of the person, criminal tendencies, experience level, and willingness to work with Mom. If a caregiver is a sociopath, as a small percentage are, having a compatible element will have little impact. Pairing harmonious elements is a big first step, but not the final decision maker in caregiver selection. Always do a criminal background check. Having video cameras, as I do, certainly helps spot mentally deranged caregivers who, for whatever reason, were able to tiptoe through the door and ace the interview. Knowing how to match elements has saved me a great deal of time and grief caused by caregiver turnover.

Having watched the interaction between my mother and her 200+ caregivers, I have been able to study closely the similar behaviors of element groups; though anecdotally so – enough that I realized there truly *seemed* to be a predictable correlation between element pairs.

My discovery regarding caregiver compatibility with my mother could be a compelling research study as the baby boomer generation draws closer to the age of needing personal care and assistance. Perhaps my observational findings might pave the way to formal research of the correlation between human relationships and Feng shui element combinations as a method to assist with matching helpers to vulnerable persons in need of understanding, supportive caregivers. For now, if you are looking to match a compatible caregiver to a loved one, an agency looking to pair caregivers to clients, or looking for a helpful person for yourself, this book promises to enlighten you to a new idea that has proven itself in my experience for the daunting task of partnering compatible caregivers with my mother.

# First Things First

## Feng Shui

*"The most important thing to understand is that feng shui is really about the energy that's surrounding you in your personal space."* --Lillian Too

The Chinese term Feng shui translates as "wind-water" in English, and relates to the energy forces around us. The goal of Feng shui is to create the perfect environment with the right energy (or chi) to produce good fortune in love, money, health, and harmony. Depending on your element, you will have auspicious vs ill-fated directions, colors, and items that when used well, can improve your life.

The purpose of this book is not to delve that deeply into Feng shui; but rather provide a simplified study of the relationships between Feng shui elements, translated to relationship balance between people.

Fire, water, metal, wood, and earth are the elements of Feng shui, each representing different characteristics and energies. Depending on birthdate, people are born to particular elements that stay with them for life. A more in depth study of the elements will follow, but first you will need to understand how to calculate kua (pronounced KWAH) numbers to determine the corresponding elements.

## Kua Calculation

*"To the extent math refers to reality, we are not certain; to the extent we are certain, math does not refer to reality." –Albert Einstein*

Before we explore which caregivers might harmonize best with your loved one, your client, or yourself, we need to understand how to calculate kua numbers in order to determine elements. Kua numbers are personal numbers calculated by birth month and year, and used in Feng shui to determine lucky directions, colors, and elements.

The calculation is simple, yet slightly different between males and females, as well as those born in January or the first half of February. Begin by adding the last two digits of the birth year to arrive at a single digit (e.g., '56 becomes 5 + 6 = 11, then 1 + 1 = 2).

If born in January or the first half of February, subtract 1 year (e.g., 1956 becomes 1955). If calculating for a male, subtract the single digit from 10, so 10 − 2 = 8. If figuring for a female, add the single year digit to 5, so 2 + 5 = 7.

The example below adds the last two digits 56 together to arrive at 11, next adding those two digits together to arrive a 2. The next step depends on gender. For females, calculate by adding the 2 to 5, arriving at 7; or for a male, subtract 2 from 10, which is 8. So a female born in 1956 has the final number of 7, while a male born in the same year has the number 8.

If NOT born in January or first half of February:

| Female Calculation | Male Calculation |
|---|---|
| **Birth Year:** 1956 = 56 | **Birth Year:** 1956 = 56 |
| **Reduce 56 to one digit:** <br> 56: 5 + 6 = 11 | **Reduce 56 to one digit:** <br> 56: 5 + 6 = 11 |
| **Reduce 11 to one digit:** <br> 11: 1 + 1 = 2 | **Reduce 11 to one digit:** <br> 11: 1 + 1 = 2 |
| **Add single digit to 5:** <br> 2 + 5 = 7 | **Subtract single digit from 10:** <br> 10 -2 = 8 |
| The kua number for a female born in 1956 is **7**. | The kua number for a male born in 1956 is **8**. |

The previous example assumes the person was not born in January or the first half of February. Let's try the example again, for someone born in January.

If born during January or first half of February:

| Female Calculation | Male Calculation |
|---|---|
| **Birth Year:** 1956 = 56 | **Birth Year:** 1956 = 56 |
| **Subtract one year from actual birth year:** 1956 − 1 = 1955. | Subtract one year from actual birth year: 1956 − 1 = 1955. |
| **Reduce 55 to one digit:** 55: 5 + 5 = 10 | **Reduce 55 to one digit:** 55: 5 + 5 = 10 |
| **Reduce 10 to one digit:** 10: 1 + 0 = 1 | **Reduce 10 to one digit:** 10: 1 + 0 = 1 |
| **Add single digit to 5:** 1 + 5 = **6** | **Subtract single digit from 10:** 10 - 1 = 9 |
| **The kua number for a female born in January 1956 is 6.** | The kua number for a male born in January 1956 is **9**. |

It is important to calculate correctly based on year, gender and whether a person's birth month falls in January or early February, because as you can see in the above examples, the final numbers are quite different, as will be the elements.

Each kua number relates directly to a specific element. The element represents the person's natural energy, as related to the world around them, personal characteristics, favorable directions, and preferences. Once you have calculated the kua number, you will be ready to discover the element and relational characteristics.

## The Five (Elements)

*His life was gentle, and the elements so mixed in him that Nature might stand up and say to all the world, "This was a man!" --William Shakespeare*

Each kua number represents a particular element. Each element corresponds to certain energy that may be in harmony with, control vs controlled by, or nurture vs nurtured by certain other elements.

Below is a table that illustrates the element related to each kua number.

| Kua Number | Element |
|------------|---------|
| 1 | Water |
| 2 | Earth |
| 3 | Wood |
| 4 | Wood |
| 5 | Earth |
| 6 | Metal |
| 7 | Metal |
| 8 | Earth |
| 9 | Fire |

Three of the kua numbers are related to earth, two each to wood and metal, and only one each for water and fire. Notice that earth people outnumber water or fire people (3:1), which will make it easier to find earth caregivers than those of water or fire – which is fine because most earth caregivers are compatible to all. If you need fire or water caregivers, and find them, be sure to retain them if they are free of emotional defect, as from my experience, water and fire have been the most difficult to find.

Also worth noting is the mild contrast I have noticed between like element caregivers with different kua numbers. Earth includes three numbers – 2, 5, and 8. Kua number 5 translates to 2, so there are really only two earth numbers: 2 and 8. I have known many earth people – no surprise since more people are earth than any other element; and have noticed personality distinctions between them, depending on their number.

Those with kua number 2 (and 5) seem more at ease with life, regardless the circumstances; while those with kua number 8 seem at times uptight and emotional, unpredictably so. The earth, itself, has different contours and makeup; so not surprising that some earth people can be consistently like warm sandy beaches, while others occasionally erupt like a volcano after a long period of silence.

The two metal numbers, 6 and 7, also seem to have slight differences, with 7 being less patient, and 6 more manipulative; though both are equally bright.

Wood kua number differences are less obvious to me, although my 4 wood mother seems more emotional than her 3 wood caregivers; yet when paired with 4 wood caregivers, the energy exchange between seems equally unstable.  I watched her interact with a 4 wood caregiver once, and the involvement  seemed more like a contest of wills than a care relationship.

Although elements of more than one kua number have basic similarities, they do seem to have minor, but notable, differences. The distinctions may be related to mental health flaws or kua number – yet seem to exist.

## Nurturing Elements

*"Be the one who nurtures and builds. Be the one who has an understanding and a forgiving heart one who looks for the best in people. Leave people better than you found them." –Marvin J. Ashton*

The five natural elements nurture and are nurtured by other elements, producing a perfect energy cycle among the elements.   Water hydrates wood. Wood feeds fire. Fire enriches earth.  Earth shelters metal.  Metal fortifies water.

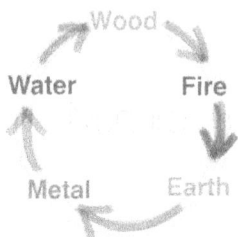

## *Controlling Elements*

*"Manipulation, fueled with good intent, can be a blessing. But when used wickedly, it is the beginning of a magician's karmic calamity."*  --T.F. Hodge

Each element has the power to control one other element. Water extinguishes fire. Fire reforms metal. Metal cuts wood. Wood holds earth. Earth restricts water.

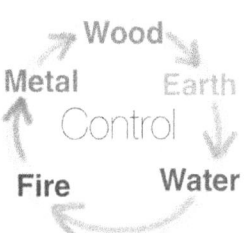

Elements usually govern other elements in a constructive manner, keeping their balance in

check; yet have the power to cause total destruction, for reason, or not.

With some understanding of how elements interact in nurturing or controlling ways, it is time to take a more in depth look at how they behave when combined. By the time you finish reading this book, you will be able to match caregiver and client elements to provide the most nurturing care your loved one, client, or yourself needs and deserves.

# Elements of Personality

There is balance in nature involving the five basic elements of water, wood, fire, earth, and metal – each playing a critical role to maintain homeostasis for our planet. Water nurtures wood, which nurtures fire, which nurtures earth, which nurtures metal, which nurtures water – a system that maintains connection with purposeful interaction.

I am not a geologist, so will not try to write in scientific terms; but I do have a layman's understanding of how the system works. Picture a mobile attached to baby's crib. Each part is connected by separate strings, allowing all parts to move together in perfect balance. If one or more of the strings become tangled or loosed, balance becomes broken, and the system no longer moves in a synchronized manner. Homeostasis is lost. Elements function in a similar manner. If one element is lacking, especially water, everything suffers.

Think of what happens during a severe drought. Trees and plants become dehydrated, and roots deep inside the dry, cracked ground shrivel, allowing the connected grass, plants, and trees to die. Perhaps an unintentional spark ignites the dried grass and trees, providing ample fuel for wildfire. The rich fire residue that would normally permeate the soil to encourage new plant and tree growth cannot penetrate the hardened earth. Nothing grows. Trace metals that rest on the soil and normally wash into and fortify streams and rivers via wind and rain become stuck in place.

The situation cannot change until heavy rains come again to moisten and soften the earth, allowing potent fire residue to penetrate, and metal particulates to wash into streams and rivers. The entire system is off-kilter, as when a string becomes tangled on a baby's crib mobile. Elements that are out of sync, or otherwise lacking, behave differently than those that are well-nourished, and the relationship between them can deviate from the intended design.

That said, when elements are properly nourished, the entire system moves in a natural circle to provide all that is necessary to create and maintain life with connection and purpose; and translates to a set of personality traits in humans that guide how we interact with the energy around us – energy that influences our comfort and preferences (e.g., auspicious compass directions we find comfortable to face, sleep in, even what colors attract us). Our personalities shift toward the element of our birthdate, and we seem drawn to or repulsed by others based on the energy that radiates between.

Think about it for a moment. Reflect on the last time you met someone new. Think about how you felt as you introduced yourself. Were you instantly comfortable? Or was there a hint of uneasiness? The energy between was either positive or negative, and probably not at all related to the way the person was dressed, or how they wore their hair. It was just *something* that either made you feel like hanging around and talking, or making an excuse to leave. That was energy. We feel energy, though we do not generally see it.

Energy between people exists. Call it what you like – familiarity, connection, in sync, out of sync, instant bond, love at first sight, good vibes, kismet, whatever. Energy moves back and forth between people, and either feels pleasant, or not; and relates directly to element compatibility. If you doubt me, check it out for yourself. The next time you are around someone you feel very connected to, or vice versa, ask their birthdate, do the math, and you will likely discover his or her element is either in or out of sync with your own.

For now, let us take a closer look at personality characteristics associated with the elements. Each one is unique with regard to attributes, purpose, preferences, and energy. For example, fire is hot, red, and charismatic, flowing up; while water is cool, blue, and soulful, with downward flow.

There is no exact profile for each element, as each can present with some differences, depending upon each person's life story; yet there are basic similarities. Wood may look strong and tall like an oak, prickly as a cactus, or delicate as a rose – all of which represent the single element of wood. There are no two people exactly alike, yet different social groups of people do share some within group similarities. Let us now move on, and learn about the different personalities.

## *Water*

What comes to mind when you think of water? Perhaps cool, clear refreshing liquid in a glass or bottle, a raindrop, a mud puddle, a deep well, a smooth pond, a bubbling brook, a lazy river, a raging river with rocky rapids and perhaps a waterfall or a dam stopping its flow, a bay, the ocean, or perhaps snow or ice, an ice cube, a frozen pond, lake, river, or waterfall. All share a similar feature – they are liquid. Yet each is unique in color, opacity, energy level, and personality.

A mud puddle is brown, murky, and still, while a stream is clear, and flows over rocks with soothing energy. Some lakes are blue. The Pacific ocean is blue. Some ponds appear black. Some bodies of water are salty, while others are fresh, relating to the different marine and green life within and around them. Water can also be polluted by raw sewage or accumulated heavy toxic metals from industry. As with people, water comes in many different forms, sizes, energy levels, and health – none exactly alike, though there are some basic things most water people have in common.

Water people are intuitive. They seem to know when things are not quite right around them; and being flexible, can move this way or that to avoid danger. Water folks can be secretive or cryptic as a defense mechanism against perceived threat. They are also kindhearted and gentle. They tend to be quiet and reserved, yet are highly creative individuals, ever-changing, and flexible. Water people have hidden potential to dominate, but actually worry more about being manipulated by others. They must balance between their fear of exploitation and hidden desire to dominate, which is not always an easy task, depending on the situation.

An unbalanced water caregiver heavy on the side of dominance is worse than an unstable client.

"Leave me alone," my mother said.

"I need to adjust your foot. It doesn't look comfortable to me," Marta said.

"It's fine.  Get your hands off me! You're hurting me!"

"Mrs. Smith, I have to do this so you'll be comfortable.  Stop fighting me."

My mother grabbed Marta's arm, pulling it away from her leg.

"Look, you goddamn bitch! I'll claw your eyes out if you don't get away from me, now!"

Marta pulled her cell phone from her pocket, and called me.

"Hi this is Marta. Stop scratching me, Mrs. Smith. Ow! Your mother is scratching me, and she won't quit. Stop it, Mrs.Smith! That hurts!"

"What is going on?" I said.

"Will you tell your mom to stop hurting me?! She just keeps hitting me!"

"Tell me what's going on!" I said.

"I'm trying to adjust her foot on the wheelchair foot pedal. It's not centered. Part of it is hanging off. Ow! And she just keeps hitting and scratching me! Stop it, Mrs. Smith!"

"I SAID, get your goddamn hands off me! You're hurting me," my mother said.

"Marta," I said, "Step away from her."

"I can't. I have to fix her foot so she'll be comfortable; but she won't stop hitting me!" Marta said.

"Marta – step away from her, and she cannot hit you," I said.

Marta stepped away from my mother.

"Marta. If she says she's comfortable, just let her be. You're making her more uncomfortable than she could've been by trying to force your idea of comfort onto her. Just go sit down, and leave her alone," I said.

"Well she won't be comfortable – and I called you to tell her to quit hitting me, and you just tell me to go sit down!" Marta said.

"Is she hitting you now?"

"No."

"Problem solved, then. What time do you get off?" I said.

"In ten minutes," Marta said.

"Ok, so just sit down, and rest until you get off. Anything else I can help you with?"

"No. I was just trying to make her comfortable." Marta said.

"I think you're making her comfortable right now. Talk to you later," I said, and hung up the phone.

*The Desire to Dominate . . .*

**Marta**, born of the element water, was loud, with fast, unpredictable movements that startled my mother. Marta's personality was contrary, seeming to enjoy the thrill of finding ways to irritate my mother (and me). She was like a rushing river full of rapids, emotionally bobbing Mom up and down like a wooden row boat against the sharp rocks. Marta would then calm down, and talk softly to my mother, like a river that relaxes to a serene, lazy flow around the bend from the rapids; and then rapids again, back and forth.

Marta's struggle for balance did not seem to resolve with my mother, so she started in on me, demanding that I use certain words when I speak, and avoid others - as an ultimatum to continue caring for my mother. My metal personality would not allow her dominance, and she finally resigned. To be quite honest, she was about to be terminated, as my mother and I had endured all that we could from her.

**Shawanda** was another water caregiver who attempted to dominate my mother through passive aggression that at times was not so passive. She began to resemble a large mud puddle full of emotional grime and parasites, polluting my mother's soul with loud splashy conversation, feeding herself from my mother's plate, and laughing like a buffoon at her protests. I watched her from the camera stand over my mother and cough into the open air, and when my mother asked her not to do that, she coughed more forcefully, followed with a laugh.

My attempts to coach Shawanda were fruitless, as she talked rather than listened, and denied every word I said, like a broken record, rewriting the facts until it would appear to an observer that

I was harassing her. Once I realized our talks were going nowhere, I terminated her from our team, and brushed the dust from my hands.

These two caregivers are classic examples of water people without balance, having unleashed the hidden desire to dominate. Both came from abused backgrounds where their personality likely shifted to survive; their unstable personalities definitely not conducive to a caring relationship.

The next two caregivers are examples of excellent balance, even in trying situations.

*Perfect Balance . . .*

**Lita's** water energy was that of an easy flowing river, clear enough to see the fishes and rocks beneath her crystal surface. She was strong and kind, never giving up on my mother, even when my mother's moods were dark and rampant. She did whatever it took to nourish my mother, cleansing her spirit until she was calm again.

When Lita enters my mother's home, she knows exactly what needs to be done, moving gracefully focused on taking my mother's blood pressure, checking her oxygen, texting the results to me, testing her blood sugar, then administering her insulin, nighttime meds, filling the pillbox, checking the oxygen tank, and many other tasks she carries out during her nightly visits.

Lita has been helping us for a very long time, and has built a solid understanding of my mother's rapid mood swings to fine tune her own inner balance to be perfectly in sync with whatever may come her way. She is a strong water person whose compassion and gentle way keeps her in balance no matter what my mother tosses her way - including the night Mom hurled her cell phone at Lita during a urinary tract infection frenzy.

**Ruthie** was like a gentle flowing stream, with a light sense of humor as one might imagine a brook skipping sweetly over rocks along the creek bed. Her energy level boundless and steady, she worked all night with my mother, and went to another full-time job the next morning. Her water soul seemed clear, pure and balanced, and her mere presence was comforting and nourishing to my wood mother who seemed like a happy tree growing by the water's edge. Ruthie was creatively skillful with my mother's moods, seeming always to know when to nourish, and when to stay quiet and wait.

Both Ruthie and Lita had ultimate control of their negative potential, as evidenced by their successful interactions with my mother, who by herself could be a major force of frustration. All four of the caregivers mentioned above were born of the water element. Two of them needed to be sucked beneath the earth's crust for rebalancing before loosing them, again. Whereas the other two lived true to their element, balancing their fears and desires nobly - nurturing my wood mother to the best of their abilities, rightfully deserving of medals for their valor in the face of my mother's difficult moments.

If looking for a water caregiver, as with any element, look for the one who shows his or her compassionate gentle self, rather than the one who is looking for someone to handle.

## *Wood*

Wood also comes in different designs, as do the people born of this element. Trees represent wood, and there are a bazillion varieties of trees, from delicate crepe myrtles to huge sequoias. All types of plant life represent wood, as do flowers – so there really is a myriad of green and brown energy to think about.

Wood people are achievers. There is no problem too great for them to handle. They are natural problem solvers – and yet, their very urge to achieve can sometimes turn to anger and verbal aggression if they become frustrated by an obstacle. They may occasionally move toward an objective without giving it much thought, as they can be impulsive decision makers if they plan too quickly.

**Nelda** was my mother's first kua 4 wood caregiver, and her personality was somewhat like a palm tree – easy, lazy, blowing in the breeze, and drop a coconut on your head if you crossed her. She was a last-minute type of person, rarely watching the time, and was usually pushing my mother in her wheelchair through the door to the doctor's office 5-10 minutes late. She was easily frustrated with my mother, and complained constantly.

**Tene** is another of my mother's wood caregivers, kua 3, still with her today. She is like a weeping willow, graceful and soft spoken. I do not recall her ever having complained about anything, and works hard, without boast. When Tene walks into my mother's home, I feel confident she will leave her better than she found her – and she always does. Tene must be an exceptional wood person as I have yet to see her anger, though I know my mother frustrates her relentlessly, at times. I think Tene is a continuous, yet silent, planner and problem solver. She makes caring for my mother look easy, when I know it is not.

**My Mother** is a classic wood personality, and I have never known her to fail at problem solving, which she does as easy as breathing. When she has an objective, better stand back and let her roll, or you will be steam rolled in the process. Her personality is stronger than Tene's, even though Tene is highly skilled at quiet manipulation. Mom has a short fuse for those who try to block her from reaching her goals, and she will not be denied what she wants.

So wood people are the natural problem solvers and achievers, mowing down obstacles in their way, with a possible side of anger for anyone who blocks their path. They are your "getter done" folks.

## *Fire*

Fire represents the color red, warmth, passion, and upward flow. Fire people are usually confident folks, and have a fairly healthy ego. Fire people at their best are generous, confident lovers of people, with no need to torch others, as they are already naturally held in high esteem. Yet they can display a sense of entitlement in certain situations.

**Athesia** was one of my mother's caregivers who treated her kindly, but would not budge to assist her unless Mom was equally kind.

"Get me a fresh glass of water, NOW!" my mother said.

Athesia looked in her direction, paused, then said, "Ask me better."

"Did you hear what I SAID?! Get OVER here!"

"And I said, ask me better."

Athesia did not tolerate rudeness, especially from a wood person who she could easily consume with one spark. She commanded kindness from my mother, or gave nothing in return. Athesia was privately known by my son and me as the ask-me-better caregiver.

Fire people are charismatic, enthusiastic, and ambitious. They love people, and many times help others without being asked; yet have an even higher regard for self. If helping others fits with their agenda, they will be first up. And they do have plans. Fire people are going places, as the upward motion of a flame indicates. They are generally quite diplomatic about getting what they want, and pretty much rule the world when water is not flowing nearby

## *Earth*

Earth represents richness, nourishment, and the mother to child relationship – hence the phrase, "Mother Earth." Earth people are generally stable and anchored, patient, reliable, and logical. They are governed by servitude, and energetic as helpers; and they will stubbornly defend those they care for.

Think of the kindest, most helpful and generous person you know. I would almost bet my paycheck the person was born of the earth element. Earth people are natural caretakers, and will always move to the front of a help-needed line. It is what they do.

I once knew a generous kua 2 earth person who took care of both his parents in his home during their final days; first one, then the other. He currently cares for his aunt, who recently also came to spend her last days in his home. I personally do not understand this high level of compassion, as caring for the dying is difficult, at best. Yet he perseveres. In his earlier days, his mother used to say, "When Dan has a nickel, everyone has a nickel" to describe his altruistic nature. Earth at its finest.

My son is also a kua 2 earth person, and pretty much a copy of his father, mentioned above, with regard to his kind and giving nature. He also opens his door to those in need, and currently offers shelter to two persons in his home. My son has opened his heart, door, and wallet to others for as long as I can remember. Another fine example of an earth person. Earth people are givers and helpers. A sad earth person would be one who had no one to care for.

**Lehana** was one of my mother's kua 8 earth caregivers. Her personality contrasts those born of kua 2 earth. She was highly emotional, self-centered, and unpredictable. She had great patience to work with Mom's mood swings, but that was her only obvious asset as a caregiver. She was routinely an hour or more late, causing other caregivers to stay until she decided to show up. She was only minimally attentive to my mother's needs, and routinely forgot to feed her.

She quit her job with the care agency for a very selfish reason. Lehana's shift was scheduled to end at 8:00 a.m. on Sunday morning. The caregiver scheduled to relieve her did not show up, so the agency let her know they were sending another caregiver who would arrive by 9:30 a.m. Lehana informed the agency she would be leaving by 8:30 a.m., and not a minute later. The agency texted me about the situation, and I requested she stay until the next caregiver arrived. Just before 8:30, Lehana transferred Mom to the bedside commode, then announced she was leaving. Fortunately I was watching via the video/audio camera, and spoke to her.

"Lehana. You can't leave while she's sitting on the commode. She needs assistance."

"Yes, I am leaving. My shift has finished, and another person is on her way."

"Lehana. The next caregiver isn't coming for an hour. She is not on her way. Please do not abandon my mother sitting on the commode."

"Yes. I am leaving now. Bye bye," Lehana said.

"Lehana! If you walk out that door, leaving her on the commode, I will report you to the State, and you'll never work as a caregiver again!"

"I know my rights, and you can't report me!"

I immediately texted the agency to stop her, or I would be reporting their employee to the State. They called and told her to at least stay until Mom was finished on the commode. So Lehana began to pressure my mother to hurry up and finish so she could leave. Of course by this time, my mother was frightened with the idea of being left alone, so she decided to stay on the commode for as long as she could. Lehana figured as much, which made her furious, and she phoned the agency.

"This is not right! I want to leave. My shift ended at 8:00, and now she's refusing to get off the commode just to keep me here! This is not right that I should have to stay and wait like this!"

By now it was 9:00 a.m., and only thirty minutes until the next caregiver would arrive. The agency told her she just needed to wait the thirty minutes so Mom would not be left alone.

"My butt is hurting from sitting so long on this commode; but I'm afraid you'll leave if I let you transfer me back to my recliner," Mom said.

"No I'm not going to leave you. I'm staying. Let me help you off the pot."

She transferred my mother back to her recliner, then out the door she went. I texted the agency, and they immediately called her. I am guessing they threatened to report her for abandonment, as she went back inside – but only after she informed the agency she was quitting her job with them for coercing her to stay. The next caregiver arrived just before 9:30, and Lehana left.

Now here was a kua 8 earth caregiver who quit her job for having to do what she caused other caregivers to routinely do when she was habitually late. She was satisfied with what she dished out, but could not deal with it the first time she was on the receiving end. Now she has no source of income because she was too impatient to work an extra 90 minutes on one occasion. She had absolutely no regard for client welfare. It was all about Lehana.

I have seen similar behavior from other 8-Earth people, which seems contrary to 2-earth's stable, patient, helpful ways – yet I am not certain whether or not the difference is related to kua number or individual mental health.

Earth people are hard workers, who excel at nearly everything they attempt to master. 2-Earth people never step in front of another also trying to reach a goal. They play fair, always giving credit where it belongs; while 8-Earth folks are not always so predictable, sometimes making stubbornly wrong decisions that only serve to hurt themselves.

## *Metal*

Metal is the source of gravity; structured, yet can accept a new form, as gold being melted to a fine piece of jewelry. Metal's energy flows inward, like a lotus flower that closes its petals. Metal's motion is determined, forceful, strong, unyielding, self-reliant, reserved, and sophisticated.

"I have therapy goals for her, today," **Veronica** said.

"That's good! Hopefully she'll be able to transfer soon," I said.

Mom had been in a hospital bed for two weeks, and was left weak, and unable to stand and transfer to the commode without a two-person assist. At home, Mom would have only one caregiver, so she needed to strengthen before leaving the hospital.

Veronica was a bright, enthusiastic metal caregiver, determined to rehabilitate my wood mother. She worked with her daily, but Mom was still not standing when it came time to discharge home. I made arrangements to have two caregivers with her for two weeks to work on mobility, and she was finally able to stand and transfer with one caregiver in a week and a half.

Veronica worked very hard to make it happen, even though met with resistance from Mom. After that goal was achieved, Veronica began to set new goals for Mom. She was met with more resistance, but Veronica did not easily give up. The more Mom resisted, the pushier Veronica became, which led to outbursts from Mom, which Veronica countered with futile debate, which eventually became ugly verbal cat fights between them.

The arguments continued day after day until Veronica resorted to cussing at Mom, progressing to the f-word in an attempt to prune her branches into submission. I talked with her about the direction the interactions had taken, and her use of profanity being inappropriate. Yet each time Mom refused her demands, she began cussing. She finally threatened to quit due to lack of compliance, so I agreed it was time for her to go.

Veronica's initial intentions were to improve my mother, but when she resorted to verbal aggression to attempt control, her intended help became abuse. Metal people set goals and follow them to exactness, where possible. They are driven and successful; definitely high achievers. However, Veronica was not in a situation where her goals could be met – as wood people also have goals, and resort to anger when blocked. Mom's intended goal seemed simply to avert Veronica's goals, so the relationship became hostile.

Metal people do not easily back down from fights, are determined, and unyielding - and Veronica was no exception. She meant well in the beginning, but was simply setting goals for the wrong element.

Had she attempted the same with an element other than wood, she would likely have been met with acceptance and appreciation, and reached her care goals, successfully.

The following chapter introduces care relationships based on element combination.

Janet Ng

# Care Relationships

Elements behave differently depending on their interaction. Fire is nourished by wood, melts metal, enriches earth, burns brighter when it joins more fire, and extinguished by water – so you might imagine the different relationship characteristics each combination creates. Fire is not comfortable with water, which reduces it to smoke and ashes; however when paired with metal, fire is on top, and can easily melt gold or silver to create a desired form. Fire adores wood that brings it to brilliance and glory, and enriches earth with residue left behind after having burned last year's crops. Fire with fire is nearly unstoppable (except by water), and rules supreme with matchless command and radiance.

Elements work together uniquely with twenty-five possible combinations, but can be altered by imbalance. During a severe drought, for instance, earth becomes dry and cracked. Trees, needing moisture and nutrients, turn brown. Even when rain comes, it may be too little too late to moisten hard, cracked earth enough to transmit adequate nourishment to the trees. People can experience emotional droughts which can alter their natural behavior. If a parched earth caregiver is with a demanding wood client, the client pulls emotionally hard on the caregiver to get needs met; but the caregiver is already drained with little or nothing to give. The wood client becomes anxious and agitated. I have seen this scenario play out in my mother's care.

One of her earth caregivers occasionally has intense personal life stressors, and her natural tendency to dote on my mother becomes temporarily subdued. When my mother pulls from her already-drained emotions, and does not get the normal attentive response, she pulls harder. She becomes agitated with the lack of emotional nurturing, blaming the caregiver, who retreats to another room until Mom finally gives up and falls asleep. Nothing much gets done that day except tugging, with no reward. By the time the water caregiver comes that night to give her insulin injection, and provide her *special water attention*, it goes without effect, as she is already too agitated to nurture.

Aside from extreme conditions, there seems a certain rhythm between elements that make relationships naturally compatible, or not.

# The Good, The Not-So-Good, and the Ultimate

*"Blondie: It's not a joke, it's a rope, Tuco. Now I want you to get up there and put your head in that noose." –The Good, The Bad and the Ugly, 1966*

My mother's primary care physician ordered home health for her which involved four initial visits from different agency representatives to begin the process. Each visit is outlined below to illustrate how my mother's wood energy related differently to each of the elements carried in by the representatives during the visits.

Visit One:

Alice (agency director) and Cate (case manager) arrived to explain available services. Mom was tired, and did not feel like talking. I asked her if it was okay for me to talk with them, and she said yes. She apologized to them for not feeling well, and I invited Alice and Cate into the next room where we could talk. I asked them both for their birth dates to determine their Feng shui element because I sensed good energy between them and Mom.

Alice's element was fire, and Cate's earth – both elements compatible with my mother's wood.

After we finished talking, they said goodbyes to Mom, which she reciprocated in a pleasant manner.

Visit Two:

The second visit entailed a health assessment by the agency's director of nursing. However when Sheila introduced herself to my mother, she was instantly met with resistance. Mom was having no part of Sheila for no obvious reason. Sheila seemed pleasant enough to me. I asked Sheila to follow me to the next room to provide whatever information she needed.

I then appealed to Mom to allow Sheila to complete the evaluation, but she refused, and became angry with me for asking. For some reason she felt Sheila was going to harm her. I went back to the other room, and apologized to Sheila for Mom's refusal, and asked what her birthdate was.

After discovering her element was metal, I reasoned that the energy between she and Mom was subpar since wood is controlled by metal, and Mom has not responded well to anyone born of metal with regard to her care. Things got worse.

Sheila got up to leave. She walked into the room where Mom was seated, and say goodbye. Mom locked eyes with her, and said,

"Get out of my house, and I don't EVER want to lay eyes on you again! GET OUT NOW!"

I had never seen my mother respond so quickly and forcefully to a metal person before. I apologized to Sheila, and she left.

Visit Three:

The following day Theresa arrived. She introduced herself also as the director of nursing. Mom smiled, and asked her to come in and sit down. The contrast in Mom's reaction to Sheila was remarkable; and the rapport between Mom and Theresa was instant. She allowed Theresa to complete the full evaluation, asked if anything else was needed, and sang "Amazing Grace" for her.

I knew Theresa's element had to be compatible with Mom's wood, so asked for her birthdate. Voila! Her element was wood – the friend element to Mom's wood. No wonder my mother was at ease with her.

I told Theresa about Mom's reaction to Sheila's metal energy the day before. Theresa told me that Sheila was no longer with the agency, which explained why her title was also director of nursing. Sheila from yesterday had apparently been with them only two weeks, and suddenly left her job within twenty-fours hours after her visit with Mom. Whatever the reason, it was abrupt; and my mother was able to perceive unpleasant energy coming from her metal element – an intuited negative truth about Sheila, and never wanted to look at her again.

Visit Four:

Pauline the Social Worker arrived. Her element was metal. Uh oh. As expected, Mom closed her eyes and turned away each time Pauline spoke to her. Pauline was respectful and kind, but my mother was having no part of her. Oddly, Mom is the one who asked for her birthdate, which enabled me to calculate her element during the interaction, and I was able to predict each turn of the visit – right up to the moment Pauline would give up and leave. I spoke with Pauline after her visit about element compatibility, and how her metal element seemed never well received by mom. Pauline suggested to try another visit in a couple of weeks, and if still no meaningful interaction, she would connect with me for whatever Mom needed.

This example with the different staff persons of the home health agency was included to show how element energy *is perceptibly* there, whether or not it can be explained by the receiver. My mother who understands nothing about Feng shui elements or energy exhibits real preference to persons with elements compatible with hers, and sometimes absolute repulsion to those with elements in control of hers.

The following chapters discuss clients of each element class and their potential relationships with caregivers from different elements. Each connection will be unique, depending on the client and caregiver combination. A fire caregiver will relate differently to water than earth, as fire is controlled by water, but it nurtures earth. So caregiver-to-client relationships will differ, depending on the elements. The chapters are divided by client, and grouped by sub-chapter descriptions of relationship qualities with each prospective caregiver element. Let us take a look to better understand how they work together.

Janet Ng

# Wood Clients

*"I drank the silence of God from a spring in the woods."* –*Georg Traki*

## *Water* Caregivers Nurture

"I'm baaack," **Ruthie** said, as she stepped over the threshold into the room.

She moved closer to my mother, who was sitting in her recliner. Ruthie clasped her hands and said,

"How's my little Snowball, tonight?"

"Well he-LLO Ruthie from Chicaaago!"

Mom's face relaxed into a smile as she looked into Ruthie's eyes.

"Where have you been?" my mother said.

"I've been WORK-ing. How have you been? Did you miss me?"

"Yes!"

Ruthie worked weeknights with my mother, and was sorely missed by her over the long, dry weekends. Ruthie is water in its purest form.

Like a warm, gentle rain in summer, she washed away all traces of the weekend drought from my mother's heart.

Caregivers born of the water element are the natural best choice for wood people – just as rain is needed by flowers, plants, and trees. I live in a city with watering restrictions due to issues with the underground aquifer that supplies water to the community. Most of the time weekly watering for a few hours is the maximum allowed to preserve water. With summer temperatures frequently in the triple digits in San Antonio, this amount is inadequate to keep many species of plants, flowers, and trees alive, let alone keep them green and lush. I lost three rose bushes, patches of grass, and the crepe myrtle leaves turned brown and fell. Yet when the temps cooled, and heavy rains fell for days during autumn, my yard reclaimed its beauty.

Wood people need water folks in their lives to stay spiritually and emotionally alive. Without them, they tend to go the way of my yard in summer, becoming irritable, needy, and morose. With water nearby, wood people are happy, vibrant, and a joy to be with as they draw comfort and strength from their necessary element.

My wood mother relied heavily on her overnight water caregiver for comfort and security. When she was having a bad time with another caregiver, she called Ruthie to make it all better with a brief chat that added instant nourishment to her soul.

Mom frequently suffers with urinary tract infection (UTI) which causes her to become agitated, sometimes aggressive, and less than a joy to be around. Ruthie was on shift with her during one of these episodes. Mom became agitated, did not recognize Ruthie, and ordered her out of the house.

Ruthie went to another room to pretend she was gone so Mom would calm down. While out of sight, Mom called Ruthie's cell phone, and told her about the awful caregiver she had banished. Ruthie listened and consoled, realizing Mom did not recognize her, and played along with the phone call. Mom finally calmed down, and they hung up.

After a few minutes, Ruthie returned to sit with Mom, only to be yelled at, as before. Mom picked up her phone, and called her again. Ruthie answered, and Mom was startled to realize the awful caregiver sitting in front of her was her dear, sweet Ruthie. My mother apologized several times, and all was well again. The natural flow of an otherwise compatible relationship was disturbed due to Mom's UTI, which added confusion and agitation to the mix.

**Lita** comes every night to give insulin injections and medications to my mother. She lives across the street, and has known Mom for many years. Lita's element is water. Over the summer, she also filled in as a regular caregiver. Mom was having another one of her UTI episodes, and did not know who Lita was, ordering her out of the house. Lita texted me about the incident, and I suggested she go home, change her clothes and hairdo, then wait for my signal to return.

I called Mom, and she told me how she threw another caregiver out of the house. I asked who it was, and she did not know. Then I asked if she wanted me to call Lita to come over and sit with her - testing to see if she knew it was Lita who just left. She said "Yes, please call Lita," so I called Lita to return to Mom.

Lita reentered this time with bright clothes and her long hair pulled up in back. She pretended it was her first time seeing Mom that day. Mom was happy to see her, telling her about the awful caregiver who just left, and they got along well the remainder of the evening.

Ruthie and Lita were often with Mom at the same time, as Lita was there to give medications, and Ruthie to spend the night. Those times appeared to be some of Mom's happiest times, as the three of them chatted, sang, and otherwise had a very sweet time together. Water was nourishing wood in double proportion, and my mother loved it.

## *Metal* Caregivers Control

Metal caregivers are usually bright, and know what is needed to keep a wood person in good shape, but can act like pruning shears to wood in a constructive or destructive manner, depending on their level of frustration. However, wood people are not at all eager to be manipulated by an enthusiastic metal caregiver, with ideas contrary to their own. They are quite content to remain unhealthy on their own terms. Thus a determined metal caregiver might easily become frustrated by a wood person not interested in the caregiver's expected compliance.

Great disharmony and chaos can result if an unyielding metal caregiver brings out the big clippers. First of all, wood people are the master manipulators of all the elements, so will rarely sit still for a well-meaning metal person who appears to be carrying a chain saw. The metal person may become angry, and walk off, which is often the case; or cut their branches with a vengeance until only a dying trunk remains. Needless to say, metal caregivers are probably not the best choice for wood people if harmony in the relationship is important.

Most metal caregivers can sense non-compliant wood energy the moment they walk through Mom's door; and she equally intuits the "controller" who enters. The other day, a metal caregiver spent less than 90 seconds with my mother before deciding to leave.

She walked up to my mother, and said, "Hi Sweetie."

The caregiver's condescending words were like a verbal challenge to my mother.

"You go sit in the kitchen," Mom said.

The caregiver picked up her cell phone, punched in numbers on the screen to dial, then said, "Pick me up, NOW." That was the end of her.

When a metal caregiver realizes my mother is a true force to be reckoned with, they usually leave immediately as this one did. When Mom senses metal character in a new caregiver, she becomes instantly gruff to ward off new attempts to control her.  Some metal caregivers come in very sweet, at first - bringing out their sword only after Mom gets cranky.  The bottom line is that metal caregivers WILL control, or leave – willingly, or by force.

## *Wood* Caregivers Befriend

"Who is that?" my mother said, as the doorbell rang.

The wood caregiver on duty pulled open the door, and said, "It's **Tene**."

"How are you doing, Tene?" my mother said.

"I'm fine, you?" Tene said.

"You coming to take care of me?"

"Yes," Tene said, and giggled.

"I had a very nice lady take care of me today. Now I've got two nice ladies here."

"That's good," Tene said with her soft, West African accent.

Tene is wood, as is my mother – a gentle, quiet wood, like a willow compared to my mother's towering crabapple tree personality. The care relationship between them reflects friendship, with Tene as my mother's confidant. They blend together as two trees in a meadow, perfectly synchronized as the breeze moves through their branches.

Wood caregivers will naturally understand the inner workings of the wood people they care for. Under normal circumstances, they should get along quite well – just as trees in the forest, and plants and flowers in the garden, they can usually coexist beautifully. Having and being a friend is important to wood people; and wood caregivers to wood clients make excellent companions. However because they feel more of a friend, they may be shy with trying to coax a client to follow a strict health schedule.

Tene is one of Mom's current caregivers, and it took her awhile to feel comfortable with suggesting Mom wear the oxygen nose cannula that my mother does not like to wear. Yet as a friend, she deeply cares for my mother, and understands her like no other element, which has motivated her to develop a friendly technique to convince Mom to comply with her health-related requirements.

Wood people are natural problem solvers. Mom had something lodged between her teeth, which was beginning to make her anxious. Tene noticed the issue, and sat beside Mom to analyze the situation. Mom explained her dilemma, while Tene listened intently. Then I watched the two of them go to work, with synchronized thought and action. Together the two problem solvers worked for about ten minutes until the issue was completely resolved. They were both focused on removing the obstacle along my mother's path to comfort.

Wood caregivers have worked out very well with my wood mother, as they seem able to blend objectives, without frustration. They understand each other, and work together in peaceful harmony.

*Fire* Caregivers  Get Cared For

"Hello, Mrs. Smith! How ARE you tonight? Got some of that Amazing Grace for *me*?" **Della** said.

My mother began to sing, with perfect pitch.

"Oh, I needed that. You always make me feel so *good* when you sing," Della said.

"Well, good! I'll sing some more, then," my mother said.

Della worked more hours with Mom than other caregivers, claiming she was lonely on her days off, sitting at home by herself. She said she was happiest when with my mother.

Fire caregivers, though dearly loved by wood people they care for, are the ones to watch in a care relationship with wood clients. Why? Because wood people are the natural caregivers for fire people, and not the other way around. Think about this for a moment. What exactly is the relationship between wood and fire when you put a log in the fireplace, blending the two elements? Fire consumes wood until it becomes a pile of ashes, having given itself totally to the fire. The word "exploitation" comes to mind.

Wood people have a great inner desire to satisfy fire people, and very much enjoy seeing their eyes light up when they do things to make the fire person happy. The fire person naturally delights in receiving from wood people – to the point of sometimes creating situations to be cared for by the wood person, such as a fire that dies down, threatening to completely extinguish if another log is not quickly added to increase the flame.

This type of relationship may be perfect in a marriage, but could lead to financial exploitation in a care relationship. I witnessed what resembled this type of interaction begin between my mother and Della. She told my mother she could not drive her anywhere because she could not afford car insurance. Next I got a call from my mother saying she wanted to give Della cash to buy car insurance. Della did not have a driver's license, let alone a car to insure. Of course my mother did not provide money for the claimed need, and Della was later discharged for trying to drive a wedge between my mother and me, lying, and insubordination.

A potential exploiter usually begins the process by attempting to isolate the intended victim from family and friends so that no one is near enough to interfere. They accomplish this through driving emotional wedges between the intended victim and others by setting up scenarios that cause the victim to mistrust or otherwise be angered with everyone close except the exploiter. They plant ideas into the victim's mind that look as though the family or friends are enemies, with the exploiter as the only true friend the victim has. If the victim is elderly with some measure of cognitive decline, it is not that difficult for an exploitive caregiver who spends a great deal of private time with the victim to succeed. Once the separation from concerned others is established, the exploiter feels comfortable to victimize.

Della was driving a wedge between my mother and me so skillfully that I did not at first recognize the red flags. Nearly every time I visited during Della's shift, Mom spoke to me with an angry tone until I left. It got to the point where I could not be there more than 30 minutes before walking out the door. She and Della seemed to have a private joke between them as they frequently exchanged glances when I spoke. It seemed like my mother was trying to impress her with the unkind words she said to me. Della did not say anything in my defense, and that puzzled me.

Della started bringing her own family members to visit my mother, and frequently arranged FaceTime exchanges between her fiancé and Mom, and often while I was there to visit. My visits with Mom were frequently dominated by Della and her fiancé. Yet I still did not understand what was happening.

Della got sloppy one night, and accidentally sent a text about me, to me, that was intended for her fiancé. The text involved accusations that seemed like I was on drugs, and that I never stayed long for visits, like I was not fit, nor cared about my mother.

When I confronted Della about the texts, she lied, and claimed she was referring to her son, not me – even though she called me by name and referred to "she," and not "he." She seemed incensed that I dared question her about it, and responded with, "I am not going to argue with you about it, take that how you want to, and this conversation is now closed." Her response to my question about the texts was translated by me as insubordination and lying, and I terminated her abruptly.

My mother's anger toward me disappeared the next time I visited her, and she has not been routinely agitated with me since Della left. I cannot say with certainty that Della was setting my mother up for exploitation, but the initial red flags were certainly present.

Two months after the termination, she knocked at my mother's door to get sympathy from her about my having fired her. My mother's memory is failing, and she no longer even recognized Della, but was upset that Della was talking to her about me. I happened to be watching the camera during her surprise visit, and I spoke to her, demanding that she leave, and not return. We will never know, thankfully, whether or not Della was truly setting my mother up for exploitation, as she was terminated before she had much of an opportunity.

Mom has had a couple other fire caregivers who behaved appropriately with her, and showed no red flags for potential exploitation – yet one was terminated for excessive absences.  The other left due to career advancement.

If you must use a fire caregiver with a wood person, keep a watchful eye, and pull out the logs if the flame goes too high.

### *Earth* *Caregivers Become Controlled*

"Mrs. Smith, are you hungry? Would you like me to fix you some bacon and eggs with crispy, crunchy toast?" **Salena** said.

"Not right now.  I want to sleep awhile longer."

"Ok, Mrs. Smith.  I'll ask you again when you wake up."

Salena is earth, the element controlled by my mother's wood element.  She intuits well how to work on my mother's terms, without argument or coaxing. She is easy-going, as earth people are, and comfortable working without strict routine, always patient to wait on my mother's timing in all aspects of her care.

Earth people are givers, by nature; and sharing their rich inner beings with wood people is one of their natural faults that can drain them, sometimes beyond repair, but they cannot resist. They are similar to potting soil that can become sterile and depleted of its nutrients from the constant draw of a hungry plant.

Wood people have needs, though - requiring both water and earth to survive. The wood person does not know how to stop pulling from a captive earth person. Whereas rain chooses when to grace the plant with its healing moisture, earth is a constant prisoner, held firmly by wood's roots, often with no escape as wood saps its strength. That said, these two elements do get along quite well, naturally – but the earth caregiver can become emotionally exhausted by the wood person, especially if the caregiver is in a depleted state to begin with, or does not have a way to recharge.

Selena has been with my mother for over a year, and is currently the only earth caregiver still there. Most of the others left because they were not fully equipped to provide very long for Mom's demanding nature.  Selena gets exhausted, but has always managed to recharge.  She has developed a repertoire of techniques to keep Mom's wood from devouring her. She thinks beyond the situation, and always manages to keep Mom's sometimes barbed  roots at bay.

"Mrs. Smith, you have a doctor appointment today. We should probably start getting ready."

"I *am* ready. Let's go."

"You have to eat your breakfast and get dressed, first."

"I'm trying to sleep. Leave me alone."

"Alright, then. How about I fix your breakfast while you rest?"

"That's a good idea," my mother said.

Selena prepared bacon, eggs, and toast, and presented it to my mother.

"Here's your breakfast, Mrs. Smith. Would you want to eat it now?"

"Can't you see I'm sleeping? Go 'way."

"We have to leave in a little while, and you still have to take your medicine and get dressed. Would you like me to feed you now?"

Mom drew her hand back, and brought it down hard on Selena's arm.

"Go 'way, you godammed bitch! I'm not going!"

Selena stepped back a minute, then walked to the other side of the room and sat down. She called me, and I suggested she cancel the appointment since by now it did not seem they could get there on time. So she did.

Mom opened her eyes about fifteen minutes later.

"You'd better get your shoes on, and take me to the doctor," Mom said.

"I already cancelled the appointment since you said you weren't going," Selena said.

"Well you'd better UN-cancel it, and get me ready."

Salena approached Mom to help feed her breakfast, and Mom slapped her, again.

"I'm not coming near you if you are going to hit me."

Salena walked away from Mom, and sat down.

"Get back over here and feed me!"

"No, Mrs. Smith. I'm not going to allow you to hit me, anymore."

"Did you HEAR MEEE!! I said get over her, NOW."

"Mrs. Smith, I'm not coming over there as long as you are yelling at me."

"You're gonna make me late for my appointment! Get over here NOW!!"

"I'm not coming near you until you speak kindly to me."

"You're going to make me late! Now get over here NOW!"

"No, Mrs. Smith, you're going to make yourself late, because the longer you talk mean to me, the longer I'm going to sit here."

Mom did not respond. She closed her eyes as if asleep. Salena remained in her chair, silently waiting – holding her ground.

Two long minutes later Mom finally spoke. Her voice was quiet and soft.

"I am sorry. I don't know why I spoke to you that way. I do want to go to the doctor. Will you help me get ready?"

"Of course I'll help you, Mrs. Smith."

Just like that, all was forgiven. Salena had skillfully shut off her nurturing supply until Mom's roots stopped twisting and squeezing.

Earth people are forgiving souls, but not fools; and my mother knew that about Salena, which is probably why she gave up to let Salena win. Mom needed her, and Salena understood that, which is why she likely refused to move until Mom agreed to play nice.

Salena takes a lot of anger from my mother. I sometimes wonder why she stays. She is a good caregiver who could get another job without effort.

She told me once, "I have a soft spot for your Mom."

I pondered her words – wondering *how could that be?* Yet it is fairly simple. Earth supports wood as a mother cares for her child, even thru the "terrible twos."

# Fire Clients

*"To poke a wood fire is more solid enjoyment than almost anything else in the world." --Charles Dudley Warner*

## *Wood Caregivers Nurture*

Fire needs wood to bring it crackling to life. If you have been comfortably in front of a wood-burning fireplace, you have seen it in action. The more wood, the bigger the flame. There is a natural bond between wood and fire, which can be exciting at its peak, and soothing as it adds a gentle light of pulsing red glow to the embers. More wood is periodically placed on the fire to keep it alive, until you are ready to put it out, or run out of wood, whichever comes first.

The relationship between fire and wood people is similar. Somewhere in a happy fire person's life is an abundant wood person, creating and sustaining the flame – a healthy wood person who continues to grow.

My uncle lives on a 16-acre ranch full of trees, and has fed his wood-burning fireplace and stove during winter for over 20 years from mere deadfall. One might think he would surely run out of wood after 20 years. That is not the case. His property remains beautifully abundant with trees of green. Why? – because for each limb that falls, another sprouts due to his vigilant care and management of his property. His wood supply is never ending, and will continue to be so as long as it is well cared for. As an interesting side note, my uncle's element is earth, which is controlled by wood, and may explain why he has been naturally compelled to provide impeccable care to his trees.

The same is true for human relationships. The wood person must be reliable and strong, always growing, in order to continue feeding a hungry fire person for any length of time – and most wood people are amazingly resilient, which is how the relationship remains a strong one, and why a wood person makes the natural best choice as caregiver to a fire client. It is possible, however, that a vulnerable, or otherwise weak wood person could become exhausted by fire's insatiable demand, and become totally used up if alone with no regrowth of precious inner resources.

This scenario might be particularly troubling if the fire person is the caregiver, struggling to make a living, while the wood person is the client with money enough to pay for care. For the wood person in the previous section, I pointed out that a fire caregiver could become exploitive; yet a wood caregiver would be unlikely to do the same to a fire person, as a wood caregiver is the giver, not the taker, in the relationship.

A relationship between a wood caregiver and a fire person makes much more sense than the other way around, as the wood caregiver will likely go that extra mile on a routine basis to make sure the fire person is safe, happy and well cared for. The fire person will never tire of care and affection bestowed by a wood caregiver. The relationship is next to perfect.

*Water* Caregivers Control

Water naturally controls fire. When the flames burn too high, or wild, they can be controlled or extinguished with water. Even out of control wildfires are eventually snuffed out after some time and effort via low-flying planes pouring huge buckets of water onto the flames. Having a water caregiver for a fire person is opposite to stimulating, and not the most pleasant time for the fire person who needs to burn brightly to stay emotionally and mentally alive – not to mention: fire does not like water. A water caregiver to a fire person is like a dark cloud that shrouds the sunlight. Unless the fire person is totally out of control, and needs restraint, a water caregiver should probably be avoided.

I have noticed an intriguing reaction between my mother's fire and water caregivers. Lita is Mom's water neighbor who stops by nightly to give insulin injections. She can silence the room merely by walking into the home when a fire caregiver is present. On nearly every visit, the fire caregiver stopped chatting with Mom, and retreated to another area of the room away from her as if on cue. The fire caregiver remained silent until Lita left, and made no attempt to converse with Lita, and spoke only when spoken to. Fire caregivers tend to distance themselves from Lita on nearly every one of her visits. When Lita left, each of the fire caregivers resumed their interactions with my mother. Lita did nothing wrong to provoke such a reaction. Rather it seemed to be fire's natural defensive instinct to retreat until Lita's water energy had gone.

Fire is naturally threatened by water. The negative interaction between a water caregiver and a fire client will be more pronounced than between two caregivers. At best, the fire client will likely be anxious having the water caregiver's energy in such close proximity for long periods of time. At worst, the fire client may completely shut down, emotionally. In my opinion, there is no good water caregiver for a fire client – unless behavioral restraint is the goal, as with Ted Bundy, the well known serial killer who was born of fire and died by fire from the electric chair. He might have been best managed by a strong water prison guard while still alive. However a normal, non-deviant fire client will not likely fare well with the restraint of a water caregiver.

## *Fire* Caregivers Befriend

Fire personalities blend well, making a fire caregiver a splendid choice for a fire client. The caregiver will have a natural understanding of the client's needs. The sum of this relationship is definitely greater than its parts, as each detonates the other, simultaneously and constantly. The growth between the two can be exponential.

Fire people tend to be charismatic, talkative, and very much enjoy being in the spotlight. Two fires blend easily to share the attention. Together, fire people are like Batman and Robin, nearly unstoppable at whatever they choose to pursue.

The agency that has provided part of the care service to my mother is owned by a fire person, and his office manager is fire. They seem to work well together; sometimes teaming up to handle me when my metal energy becomes too demanding and unyielding. If I become disenchanted with one of them, the other joins the process to reframe my point of reference, as fire reforms metal.

On one occasion, I was not happy with the owner, whom I had not yet met in person, for not meeting the demands of my unrealistic expectations for my mother's care. I stopped communicating with him, altogether. I was new to the caregiving world, and had preconceived notions for how the process ought to work. My attitude was not conducive for a good working relationship, and the two of them set out to help correct the error in my thinking.

After vowing that I would not speak to the owner again, the manager contacted me to set up a one on one meeting with her to discuss the future of my mother's care relationship with the agency. Although reluctant to commit, I agreed to allow her to come to my home for a meeting. When I opened the door, she was standing there with the owner. Two fire people standing at my door was enough to melt my metal energy to a puddle on the floor. What else could I do but invite them both in.

Rather than use their fire power to destroy what was left of the business relationship, they worked together to improve the relationship by reframing how I looked at things until I was ready to understand how things truly needed to work for my mother's best interest. They reformed my sword into a ring of gold, and I have held the owner in high esteem ever since.

Things could have gone badly if they had simply brought out the blow torch, and blasted me with ultimatums – as fire people are highly capable of doing; but instead they used their energy to turn the relationship into workable energy between us. I recognized their constructive effort, and wisely yielded to it for my mother's sake. We have gotten along well since that day; and I do recognize from time to time when they are handling my metal rigidity. They work exceptionally well together, as fire with fire.

Having a fire to fire care relationship can work equally well. The two will help each other, entertain one another, and influence one another in the relationship as no other like elements can. As long as both client and caregiver have good character, it is likely a marvelous match. Of course, having Ted Bundy's fire in the mix could be a disastrous combination, so make sure the fire caregiver is not deviant by watching and listening through cameras for a while.

## *Earth* Caregivers Get Cared For

Earth caregivers draw much from vibrant fire people – just as soil becomes enriched from fire residue after burning grass or crops. A favorite color of earth people is red, which represents fire, and they can spend many a contented hour gazing at an open flame of a fireplace or campfire as it soothes their inner being.

Earth does not necessarily do anything for fire, save being the home of the wood element that feeds fire. The relationship is very unlikely to be exploitive, as it can be between a fire caregiver and wood client. In that relationship, fire threatens to go out if more wood is not supplied – but there is no enticement from earth to get something from fire – it simply accepts what fire gladly provides. The care relationship is thusly in reverse, as it is fire that naturally provides to earth, and not the other way around. That does not mean an earth caregiver will not care for a fire client – he or she definitely will, as earth people are natural helpers to any element, but especially to fire that nourishes their spirit. Yes, an earth caregiver will happily be in devoted servitude to an ailing fire person perhaps as payback for what fire naturally does for earth.

My son spent quite a bit of time with my mother's late husband before his passing. Raymond was fire, and my son, earth. Oh how Raymond lit up when Douglas came to visit, and Douglas seemed not to tire of long conversations with Raymond.

Raymond loved to fish, and Douglas took him fishing and camping, on occasion. Raymond fell victim to cognitive decline during his last few years, and Douglas seemed an especially sensitive comfort to Raymond during some of his darker days. Douglas' kind, caring earth element was able to soothe Raymond with conversations about fishing, which usually led to a show and tell of Raymond's newest rods and reels, which on occasion inspired Ray to gift his step-grandson with one of his treasured items – his fire element enriching Douglas' earth. They shared a special bond that Raymond shared with few.

Even though fire is the natural giver to earth, earth is the natural giver to all, which makes this a very rewarding care relationship for both. Earth is well-grounded, while fire flows upward, so that both elements pull toward the middle for an accurate measure of balance. Earth controls the water element fire fears, and fire rewards earth generously.

## *Metal* Caregivers Become Controlled

A metal caregiver will be controlled in one way or another by a fire client, and perhaps not comfortably so. Fire almost always has the upper hand with metal; hence the ability to melt silver and gold, or weld steel into a different form. The metal caregiver will not win at getting a fire person to take unwanted medicine or submit to unwelcome therapy. The caregiver may wield the sword, but the fire person simply melts it with flames of anger or skillful manipulation. This is not a good care relationship if the fire person is uncooperative with needed treatment.

Raymond was hospitalized on several occasions during his last couple of years, and was an uncooperative patient, though years before had been a model patient. Cognitive decline changed him, and he no longer felt safe in the confines of a hospital. I tried my best to console him, but he only begged me to take him home, or ignored me because I could not. His attempts to manipulate me eventually  weakened, and he simply resigned to punish me with silence, which effectively hurt my metal feelings – an element he had little trouble handling just a few years earlier.

During my weekend visits to my mother and Raymond's home, he never failed to  have jobs for me  -  finding a lost item, helping him research his latest interest, taking him shopping, taking a walk, teaching him how to use his newest technology purchase after assistance with assembly, or simply listening to him complain about my mother.  He usually dominated my visits, which was okay with me, as I was there to help where I could.  He was a fire person trying to hang onto to self-esteem, and my element was there to help as often as I could make the three-hour drive from Houston to San Antonio.

Having a metal caregiver may not be totally bad for a weakened fire client who is struggling to maintain dignity. The metal caregiver who yields to  fire energy may help bolster the fire person's ego.  However, the metal caregiver may pay the price through busted self-esteem, or stress-related illness.

Metal people have a tough time saying "No" to fire people, allowing the other to twist them into uncomfortable emotional positions. The metal person is intimidated by the fire person's flame; and may either melt beneath the heat of the torch, or leave the relationship to avoid total meltdown.

Raymond did not control me, destructively, but rather intently in a positive manner. Perhaps I would have become exhausted as his caregiver on a daily basis, but my frequent weekend visits were not enough to cost too much energy loss for me. I recall my mother telling me, just before I moved to San Antonio, "Raymond said he's so glad you are coming because he says you'll go on walks with him, and make me be nice to him." My mother was beginning some mental decline at that point in time, and was not always the easiest person to be with; and Raymond seemed to catch most of her mood swings, and hoped I would somehow bring relief. I did have some power to help, as my metal element controls my mother's element of wood.

In our situation, metal helping fire was good for Raymond, and non-destructive for me; however, in day-to-day care, it would likely be more taxing on the metal caregiver.

# Earth Clients

*"My beloved is the sun, and I am the earth that thrives only in her warmth." --C. L. Wilson*

## *Fire* Caregivers Nurture

The very best caregiver an earth person can have is someone born of fire. Fire enriches earth. Earth folks love fire people, and will most likely cooperate with care. They simply enjoy having their fire nurturer nearby for fellowship and warmth.

The earth client is stable and balanced, while the fire caregiver is charismatic, daring, and fun for the earth client to be with. The fire caregiver will inspire the earth client to do his or best. The relationship is therapeutic and comfortable for both. The fire person is always delighted to give, and earth person content to receive from one who knows him or her so well.

President Ronald Reagan was born of the fire element, while his wife Nancy was born of earth. According to an article in the Chicago Tribune, written June 6, 2004 by Michael Kilian,

"Ronald Reagan's marriage to his second wife Nancy was as close and strong a partnership as the White House has ever seen."

Although Nancy's earth cared for President Reagan's fire during his illness, and beautifully so according to the article, I am convinced the reverse would also have been true. Earth and fire are very good together, as there is no control in the relationship, only nurturing. Fire nurtures earth, and earth nurtures all elements. This seems definitely a care relationship to seek out.

## *Wood* *Caregivers Control*

Wood people can be manipulative, especially with easy-going earth folks who they control. Their roots run deep into the earth, twisting in whatever directions and configurations they desire. Earth is uncomfortable denying a wood person, and will generally go along to get along, as earth craves stability and peace. An earth child to a wood parent will likely be golden as he or she will undoubtedly obey orders without resistance, even though feeling resentment underneath. An adult earth client may not be as compliant, but after debate, the wood caregiver will usually come out on top.

Wood cares for earth. Why would it not? Without earth, most wood species could not survive. Yet wood calls the shots, and has little argument from earth, captive beneath its feet. Earth has no choice but to supply whatever wood pulls from it, possibly until there is nothing left to give.

That said, wood people do make good caregivers – better for fire people whose element they nurture, but also possibly for earth people, as they are determined problem solvers. I probably would not choose a wood caregiver for an earth client only because they may be too pushy and manipulative, resulting in too much drain on the earth person's already weakened reserves.

My mother adores her grandson, my son – but I can recall a time when she pulled too much from him until my metal element that controls her wood element intervened. We shared an apartment just north of Houston. My son was in high school. Nearly every day when he got home from school, she requested that he take her places, and he did. However it got to the point where he was refusing social engagements to drive her around, and he could not tell her "No." I finally stepped in, and told her, myself, which was not a good scene, but at least she loosened the grip of her roots so he could breathe.

She loved him dearly, and did not even realize how great was her pull. Once she did, however, she was able to back off, and let him have his space.

Earth people have a hard time refusing a wood person. A care relationship between the two, with earth as the client might not be compatible for this reason. Yet I am sure there may be a strong earth person somewhere who can handle the drain, and has learned to stand his or her ground when wood's pull becomes too great – which is the only way this relationship could work. Wood people are determined, though, so it could be a constant struggle for the earth client to maintain his or her position.

### *Earth* Caregivers Befriend

Earth people naturally gravitate toward one another. They get along in an easy, relaxed way better than any other like-element combo. Earth people rarely disagree with each other, at least not openly, as they are naturally kind, and do not wish to hurt each other's feelings. The main reason they do not argue is because they are so much alike. They enjoy the same things, think alike, and are other-focused. They put each other first.

I once knew an earth-earth couple that honestly had no arguments until just before their divorce, which was triggered by the wife's infidelity. When her husband stumbled onto the affair, her deepest regret was not for having the affair, but rather for how badly he was hurt when he found out. The husband gave her another chance, as she promised to be faithful from that point forward. She was not, and they finally divorced.

Earth people would almost rather die than hurt another individual. That does not mean that all earth people are perfect, as illustrated above – but they certainly have kind hearts that do not intend to inflict pain on others. They genuinely care about people of all elements. It is interesting to note that the wife's element was 8-Earth, and the husband 2-Earth. I mention this only because the 8-Earth wife was unpredictable and more self-serving in the relationship, while the 2-Earth husband was predictable and caring enough to give her another chance.

The same man gravitated to another earth lady, following the divorce, but this time she was a 2-earth. Their similarities are uncanny, their temperaments identical, with each putting the other first in all matters – a true demonstration of quid pro quo.

This is generally a smart match for a care relationship as earth people tend to be like-minded, and enjoy many of the the same things especially if they share the same kua number. The caregiver will go to great lengths to ensure the client's well-being, and the client will likely reciprocate so the caregiver loves the job.

## *Metal* Caregivers Get Cared For

The earth person will be more in tune with what the metal caregiver's needs are than vice versa in this relationship. Metal caregivers are bright, knowing what needs to be done in even the most complicated care plan; however their lack of tolerance for stress will have the earth patient trying to care for them, which can, in turn, increase the stress level for the earth patient. This occurs because earth is the natural caregiver for metal, and not vice versa. The metal caregiver truly cares about the earth person, but earth's instinct to care for metal will dominate, making the caregiver the "cared for." If the care plan is such that only companionship is required, this would be an acceptable scenario – especially if the client has a need to have someone to care about. But if the client has serious needs, it's better to use a different element than metal.

I have found this to be true in my own life, as a metal person – especially with my earth son. I would certainly like to think that I have been, and still am, a good mother figure to him; and am sure he would validate my claim. However, even when I am helping him, he always manages to help me more.

There is nothing wrong with a metal person caring for an earth client, as the client will likely receive top-notch care from a bright caregiver born of metal. The earth client will also offer a great deal to the caregiver in terms of cooperation, validation, and kindness. The earth client will not be demanding or exhaustive; and the metal caregiver will always have the best intentions for the person born of the element that nurtures them.

*Water* Caregivers Become Controlled

Pairing a water caregiver to an earth client can work, even with earth being the one in control, as earth people have a high regard for all elements, and would not, under normal circumstances, try to confound a water caregiver. Also, the water caregiver, being the controlled one, would have respect and hold the earth client in high esteem, consulting with, rather than dictating to the earth client. So yes, this duo gets a thumbs up in spite of earth being the one in control – translated that the earth person will have comfortable control over his or her own care plan with the water caregiver respectfully providing.

One of Mom's earth caregivers quit over a misunderstanding between she and myself. The situation was resolved, and she soon came back to work. While she was away, she called on Lita, whom is water, to assist with resolving the matter. Lita's water was influenced by the caregiver's earth element, and Lita had a soft spot for her, unable nor wanting to tell her "No." So Lita approached me about the situation. My metal element nurtures Lita's water element, so I listened to what she had to say. Before the end of the day, I contacted the earth caregiver, whose earth element cares for my metal element. Her earth told my metal everything it needed to hear to resolve the situation, and move forward.

Lita's water element, controlled by the caregiver's earth element, worked well to help get her job back. The earth caregiver's control of Lita's water element was a positive outcome for both – and Lita was happy to oblige, creatively approaching her  metal friend for help.

A water caregiver for an earth client can work well, as earth gently influences the water caregiver to provide what is needed, without undue pressure or restraint.

Janet Ng

# Metal Clients

*"The earth that holds treasures manifold in secret places, wealth, jewels, and gold shall she give to me; she that bestows wealth liberally, the kindly goddess, wealth shall she bestow upon us!" –Atharda Veda*

## *Earth Caregivers Nurture*

Earth caregivers are like kava-kava to metal people, soothing their inner spirit completely – so absolutely the best choice to match perfectly with metal people. Earth caregivers are easy-going, giving, and will relax even the most uptight metal person just by being there. They have a soft touch as helpers, and will create a very potent healing atmosphere.

My son, sister, and uncle were each born of earth, kua 2, and have the same calming effect on my metal element. When I am stressed out, I can go to any one of them and find peace and rest. I cannot count the phone calls where my metal vented its stress nonstop onto their listening ears, and by the end of the conversation, I was more relaxed than had I drank wine. I am so fortunate to have three caring earth people in my life.

Metals such as silver and gold are created in and of the earth, so the saying, "she's as good as gold" certainly depicts the earth caregiver's influence on a metal person. The earth person will nurture the metal person to Nirvana. Yes, yes, yes for this winning combination.

## *Fire* Caregivers Control

This is going to be short: Not No, but Hell No. Coming from myself as a metal person – we do not like to play with fire – at least not when we are on the receiving end. Fire caregivers have the skill and sometimes devious desire to melt and reform a metal person to their desired shape, which is stressful to the metal person. Metal people do not even like the color red – so not a good match at all. Just say no. It would be like Donald Trump, who is fire, taking care of Mother Theresa, who is metal.

## *Metal* Caregivers Befriend

Metal persons can get along, although there could be competition between them like two double-edged swords, with the sharpest blade being the victor. Care situations should not become power plays, so this might not be the best match – especially between different metal numbers (6 and 7). Two 7s may get along, or two 6s, but don't mix the numbers to avoid the clanging of swords. The same number metals think more closely alike, and may blend better, and hold the other up – that is, stick with the same metal types (gold with gold, and not silver and gold, as gold may tend to look down on silver).

I once worked with a 6 metal (I am 7), and we got along up to a point. I was thrown into a position as his supervisor – a job he had also applied for. He did not miss an opportunity to take potshots at me, constantly challenging me to mental duals. I could see it was never going to end, and made a creative metal move to put him in the position he so desired, and get relief for myself. When it came time to write the next grant, I wrote his name, instead of mine, as manager, then created a new data management position with my name attached. My earth boss's eyebrows raised a little when reviewing the draft.

"You don't want to manage the program anymore?" He said.

"It's not that I don't want to manage it, but with the new requirement to automate our data, you're going to need someone to coordinate that – and, well, you know I'm the right person for the job."

My boss paused for a moment; his eyes focused on the document before him.

"I think you're right. You are the best person to manage the data system development. But what about Larry? Do you really think he's the right person for the job you have now?"

"Unless you have someone else in mind, yes I think he can handle it well."

It was a done deal. Larry was happy, and I was happy. The creation of the new position for myself was the start of a career direction I have not regretted. As an aside, my boss was born of earth – the very element that nurtures metal. I wonder if the outcome would have been different if he were born of fire?

In summary, two metal persons might be a good choice, or not. My cousin is 7 metal, like myself; and we get along quite well. If two metals are mismatched, be sure to keep an eye out for power struggles. If none, the relationship might work well between two bright, persevering metal folks.

## *Water* Caregivers Get Cared For

Metal people have a soft spot for water people; so having a water caregiver for a metal person can work, as long as a complete role reversal does not result. The goal is for the caregiver to look out for the client, and not the other way around; or the water caregiver may, without even realizing it, become too needy for the metal person, when the metal client is the one who should be needy in the relationship. Metal people are strong, however, and may actually enjoy a *giving* relationship – yet may also become resentful for lack of turn about.

My second marriage ended due to an unbalanced relationship of a metal giver and a water taker. If this relationship had been a care relationship, rather than marriage, I the client would likely not have received the necessary care. Here is an example from my marriage.

When Brett was ill, I was at his side, bringing him medicine, chicken soup, and a cool cloth for his head. When I was sick, I got my own medicine, food and comfort. A scenario such as this would not work very well in a care relationship.

However my mother's water helper Lita has always been extra helpful to me – so perhaps the amount of help a  metal client receives from a water caregiver depends on the purity and balance of the water caregiver.  My ex-husband was not the most balanced person, often giving in to his desire to dominate; whereas Lita's water seems very well-balanced.  Keep an eye on this element combination until you are sure the client is getting the necessary care.

## *Wood* Caregivers Become Controlled

Metal caregivers are not advisable for wood clients; however the reverse can work quite well. Wood people are naturals at giving care, and will certainly dote on the metal person's needs, as well as wants.  The wood caregiver will defend the metal person to the last ounce of strength, so there is great safety for the metal client who is fortunate to have a competent wood caregiver.  It is not as good a relationship as with an earth caregiver, but it's pretty darned good.  Since the metal person has the reigns, he or she will likely guide the care, and the wood caregiver will probably be happy to comply.

My personal experience was being a metal child cared for and raised by my wood mother. We were like best friends most of my life until she started to decline over the past couple of years. She was always there for me, my mentor, confidant, problem solver, and way maker. She spoiled me more than necessary, and always found a way when there seemed no way to make things right for me.

My first memory of using my metal to manipulate her occurred inside a corner store, near the checkout. I was three years old, and wanted the Hershey's bar that was shelved at eye level to my three-year-old wonderment at the counter.

"Mommy," I said, "may I have that chocolate bar?"

"No you don't need any candy today."

"Please, Mommy – please can I have it?"

"I said, no."

My little metal brain churned to think of the words to convince her to let me have the chocolate bar.

"Mommy – if you let me have the chocolate bar, then when I grow up, and I'm your mommy, and you ask me for chocolate, I will give it to you."

My mother looked at me, laughed, then reached for the chocolate bar, and handed it to me. From that day forward, I understood the process of getting from my mother what I desired, and cannot recall a further failed attempt. The strings of her heart were wrapped securely around my fingers, and still are to this day. My metal element does not work well in reverse with her wood element -  at getting her to do the things she needs to do for herself; but if I turn it into desire, to "Do it to make me happy," she generally complies. Her caregivers have seen this in action, and frequently call me to talk her into taking her medicine when she will not accept it from them.

"Mom," I say, "I'm so tired, and need to get some sleep for work tomorrow; but I won't be able to sleep knowing you didn't take your medicine. Please do it for me."

Only out of concern for my well-being will she finally take her pills, and always asks me, if I feel better. However, she nearly always avoids me when she does not want to comply with taking medications because she knows my patience is thin, and my fuse even shorter – and if reversing roles does not work, I become frustrated, and resort to demanding she take it, which never works, and only serves to raise both our blood pressures. As a caregiver to her, I am not well-equipped with the patience required to help her do the right thing. Yet in the reverse, she has always been a very good caregiver to me. So yes, a wood caregiver for a metal person can be a smart choice, as the metal client will benefit from the wood caregiver's special attention, and be happy to be on the receiving end.

Janet Ng

# Water Clients

*"You are me, and I am You - what is the difference between us? We are like gold and the bracelet, or water and the waves." –Sri Guru Granth Sahib*

## *Metal* Caregivers Nurture

Add copper, zinc, and iron to water in trace amounts, and you've got some healthy stuff. Metal people are not natural caregivers, since so independent – yet water people are independent, as well, making the match a good one. Water people do not require a great deal of emotional support, and thrive on the trace amounts provided by the metal caregiver.

The relationship works out great as long as the metal person isn't toxic like arsenic, polluting the water. More times than not, a metal person is exactly the right match for the independent water client, as metal in proper amounts fortifies water, making it a more potent resource.

I was once married to a man born of the water element. The relationship worked well for him, as my metal element nurtured and spoiled him. I was his best friend. The reverse was not true, however, and the marriage ended because I was getting minimal in return. Care relationships differ from marriages in that the caregiver is paid to provide care, and doesn't expect quid pro quo. A metal caregiver will nurture a water client, without expecting anything more than a paycheck in return.

Lita and I get along very well, and make a great team as we coordinate my mother's care. In all the time I have known Lita, we have never had a disagreement over Mom's care. I have entrusted her to manage the medications as I know her water element cares greatly for Mom's wood element. It is a positive element circle with my metal caring for Lita's metal, which in turn cares for Mom's wood. I assist Lita however I can, and she knows I am there for her. Anytime Lita needs time off, I am ready to cover for her.

Metal to water is a very good helping direction between elements, and an excellent choice for a care relationship.

*Earth* Caregivers Control

Earth is a caring element to all elements, and a water client is no exception. Earth controls water in that it has boundaries or embankments that surround water like a security blanket. Earth simply keeps water from overflowing its banks, keeps it safe from flowing out of control. Earth people have the natural ability to keep creative water people grounded and balanced.

My water ex-husband frequently gravitated to my earth son when he was upset about something, or needed to talk. He respected my son's point of view. The connection between them was predictable. Brett always walked away from their interactions uplifted and calm. Douglas' earth energy is stable, and he has a calming effect on people of all elements; yet has particular influence on water people whose element is guided by earth.

My son confided to me that Brett was somewhat intimidated by him. Although I do not know if that was so, I noticed that Brett never antagonized my son, and held him in high regard. Perhaps my son's earth energy felt from Brett's water energy something I did not see from my metal vantage point. Brett was significantly accommodating to my son, so perhaps Douglas was correct.

An earth caregiver will likely have the same calming effect and be held in high esteem by a water client. Earth is a kind, stable provider, and a water client will probably feel secure within the safety of earth's care. The water client will likely be compliant with the earth provider's care plan. With earth as the caregiver, even in the controlling role, the relationship can work.

## *Water* *Caregiver Befriend*

Water can easily blend and flow with added water. No problem at all. When the stream meets the river, or river spills into the ocean, it is a smooth blending transition. These two will get along well, and nurture each other in a most advanced quid pro quo manner; sharing inner nutrients in the best possible way.

They are both creative. They also both have a hidden desire to dominate, and fear of being dominated – so as long as both are balanced, the relationship will work well. Yet if either of them has inner balance issues, there could be strain. Yet if both client and caregiver are fairly balanced, the relationship can flow like a sparkling stream.

## *Wood* Caregivers Get Cared For

Water nurtures wood like nothing else can, and having a wood caregiver is no exception. The water person will nurture the heck out of a wood caregiver without even noticing the roles have been reversed. It is not a bad thing, either – as water likes to quench thirst, and wood surely likes the drink. This relationship can keep  a wood caregiver happy in his or her work, while soothing the water persons need to nurture – as water gives its blessings as it wills, not being manipulated into it.

A few years back, before my mother began to suffer cognitive decline, she was helpful to Lita and her family by inviting Lita to help her with house cleaning and other chores, paying her, in exchange. Lita was happy to accept the small jobs for two reasons – she was grateful to earn extra cash, and she loved to help my mother.  Mom was in a position to help Lita, which allowed Lita to assist Mom.  They got along very well helping each other with Mom being the initiator.

Care relationships can have the same positive potential with wood helping water.  The water clients receive, but also give to the wood caregivers they adore.

## *Fire* Caregivers Become Controlled

A fire caregiver is controlled by only one element – water, and water will definitely have the upper hand in this relationship. Water can control fire, or completely extinguish it, depending on the circumstance or the water person's intentions. Water is readily used to saturate wildfires, and though it sometimes takes some time to flatten the flames, water eventually wins, though fire can do plenty of damage to other elements along the way.

I recently drove from San Antonio to College Station, along the Brazos trail, and saw plenty of evidence of the devastation fire can do before water finally ended the fury. There are miles and miles of skeletal trees where a rich forest once was, bludgeoned by a summer wildfire. However, if water is always near the flame, as a water person being cared for by a fire caregiver, the fire caregiver will likely remain subdued. In fact a fire caregiver who is not already out of control yields readily to a water person with great respect and honor.

It is sometimes better for the person being cared for to have the upper hand, than that of the caregiver, and definitely in this case. That is, having a water caregiver for a fire patient might be uncomfortable for the fire patient, but in the reverse, it is okay for the patient. However, if the water person is too restrictive, putting out even the hint of light in the fire caregiver, it might be too much stress on the fire caregiver to continue the relationship. Remember, controlling elements can manipulate constructively or destructively.

Janet Ng

# Caregiver Interviews

*"I present myself to you in a form suitable to the relationship I wish to achieve with you." –Luigi Pirandello*

Applicants are usually on best behavior during an interview. They may be nervous, yet their intention is to project a favorable persona and skill set to get hired. I do not apologize for saying that caregivers come in all shapes, sizes, intelligence levels, skill levels, and experience levels. My mother has had caregivers who were, or had previously been, paralegals, retired teachers, musicians, chefs, hair stylists, nurses, physical therapists, waitresses, bankers, college students, Ph.Ds., babysitters, dog walkers, criminals, medical assistants, certified nursing assistants, caregivers, or no real job experience at all. Some spoke clear English, some not-so-good English, some Ebonics, some several languages, and some barely spoke at all.

They arrived to the interviews dressed all different ways from scrubs to dresses, to jeans and hoodies, to African garb, to ghetto low-rider hips that clearly showed butt crack when bent forward, to shorts that showed it all.

About four in ten applicants actually showed for the interviews, leaving me to wonder why the no-shows bothered to request an interview. For those who showed up, I was interested first and foremost to the manner in which they greeted my mother, if at all, and whom they chose to speak with during the visit. Seriously, some applicants walked in, ignored my mother completely, and spoke directly to her caregiver when it was Mom who made the final hiring decisions.

I usually attend the interviews remotely via the installed video cameras because I work full-time and schedule them during my lunch breaks. I study body language and interaction with my mother. Remember people show their very best, though not necessarily their worst, during the interview – so if an applicant makes little or no attempt to interact with Mom during the interview, I do not expect them to pay much attention to her, if hired.

Some caregivers who have worked with my mother earn their pay well by focusing on her needs, engaging her, and bringing out the best in her. Others choose to sit away from her in another room, separated by a wall, occupying their time with phone in hand, or nap until she calls out to them. Mom sleeps most of the time when she has caregivers who spend their time separated from her vision field. However, with caregivers who engage her, she stays awake, has long talks with them, and has a good time during their shift. If an applicant does not bother to make eye contact with her, I predict she will be the one to sit in another room ignoring Mom while on the job, and I have usually been spot on. Needless to say, those applicants no longer get past the interview.

Watch out for applicants who call the client "Sweetie," especially if their element naturally controls the client's element  If your loved one calls you "Sweetie," it is fairly safe to interpret as a term of endearment. When a stranger calls you "Sweetie," you are likely being condescended to – and when an applicant refers to my mother as "Sweetie" when first meeting her, she may be testing the waters to determine Mom's level of submission.

Caregivers who attempted to control, handle or manage my mother on the job generally started initial interview greetings with, "Hi, Sweetie." The term quickly faded when they came to realize my mother was not a submissive bimbo on sedatives whom they could easily manage. That is usually when the ill-hired metal caregivers pulled out their swords, or headed for the door.

The best caregivers I have hired were attentive to Mom from the start; greeting her directly, talking to her directly, smiling often at her with an abundance of eye contact. The caregivers had questions to ask about the job, and easily built a rapport with her. That said, acing an interview may be good indication of an excellent caregiver, but not always the best indicator of a good caregiver *match*, as sometimes misaligned elements can initially coexist, but may be unable to continue once personal characteristics emerge on the job.

I have seen this happen many times – a top notch caregiver with a contrasting element who presented beautifully at the interview, yet failed on the job due to incompatibility, and either quickly resigned, or was terminated for inappropriate behavior with my mother.

In my experience with over 200 caregivers, I've learned to completely avoid applicants whose elements control my mother's energy. Issues unrelated to compatibility can still emerge due to initially masked mental health issues or unchecked criminal history – but the chances of match failure are far less when beginning with compatible elements.

Watch for red flags during the interview, as they generally become more pronounced on the job. An old Chinese proverb related to marital relationships says, "Before marriage, keep both eyes open. After marriage, close one." This fits with caregiver relationships, as well. Pay close attention to red flags during the interview. Once hired, be tolerant of small mistakes.

I recently interviewed an applicant over the phone who sabotaged her chance at an in-person interview after she inadvertently divulged how she managed to get full control over her last client's finances. What? She was trying to impress me with how well she cared for her last client. Within her list of what she did for the client was, "and I took care of her bills and finances as I was her financial power of attorney." What?

I waited until she finished her presentation, then asked how she came to have power of attorney over the client. She explained that the client's son had durable power of attorney for health and finances, but did not really care about the client, and threatened to put her in a nursing home.

So she talked to the client, and got her to agree that her son should not be in control of her finances. She said the son also refused to increase her pay when she clearly deserved more. She got an attorney, and was able to convince the court, with solicited help from the client, that she cared more for the client, and should be the one in charge of her finances.

Red flag! Both eyes open here! Neurons front and center! I took a deep breath, and then painted my mother in the worst possible light to her in order to allow her to be the one to back out, first.

It worked, and she said she was concerned about the pay rate, and all the care my mother needed seemed more than she realized, and would need to think about it. Big sigh of relief. However, she then said perhaps she could meet my mother, and if they got along well, she might be willing to work for the advertised pay rate.

I told her I would give her a call about a possible meeting. Not! I got a visual of her meeting my mother to see how easy it might be to manipulate her as she may have done with her previous client.

This scenario was fairly easy to flag, yet some are not as obvious. That said, the guidelines that follow will help you spot red flags, as well as green lights, or applicant pluses.

The following two tables will assist you during an interview. The first table shows each role by element to correspond with the second table of roles and things to look for during the interview.

If the client is wood, and the applicant metal, for example, the caregiver role, according to the first table, is "Controls Client."

The second table then illustrates what to look for during the interview according to the applicant's element *role* – nurturer, nurtured by, controller, controlled by, or best friends.  On the second table, the row of interest would be the one labeled "Controls Client."  For this example, a red flag might be, "Client seems tense." A green light might be, "Applicant answers questions asked, and does not answer a question with a question."

Although the green lights and red flags in the table are important to any interview, they are critical indicators between elements because element relationships are fairly predictable, and when they do not play out as expected, there could be other factors in the applicant's personal life or mental health that have altered his or her ability to have a good relationship with the client.

If the natural energy is not present between two elements that *should* be there, it could be a warning of a negative match, in spite of the element normally being a compatible one.

For a quick review of element roles, see the first table on the following page.

**Caregiver Element Roles**

| Client Element | Nurtures Client | Best Friends | Controlled By Client | Nurtured by Client | Controls Client |
|---|---|---|---|---|---|
| WOOD | Water | Wood | Earth | Fire | Metal |
| FIRE | Wood | Fire | Metal | Earth | Water |
| EARTH | Fire | Earth | Water | Metal | Wood |
| METAL | Earth | Metal | Wood | Water | Fire |
| WATER | Metal | Water | Fire | Wood | Earth |

After determining the caregiver's role, use the following tables to see red flags and green lights by caregiver role during an interview with the client. Note: The client should be present during the interview to see the the element combination interaction.

# Interview Green Lights and Red Flags

## Caregiver who nurtures client:

| Green Lights | Red Flags |
|---|---|
| Applicant makes frequent eye contact with client; Applicant smiles frequently at client; Applicant listens attentively to client; Applicant focuses more on client than others in room; Applicant quickly builds rapport with client. | Little to no eye contact between applicant and client; Client does not smile during interview; Applicant and/or client seems uncomfortable; Interview process seems awkward or slow; Applicant tries to over-impress others in the room. |

## Caregiver who befriends client:

| Green Lights | Red Flags |
| --- | --- |
| Applicant and client notice similarities about each other; Interview is more like a good conversation than a formal interview; Applicant and client appear to genuinely like each other; Client seems relaxed, as does applicant; Light-hearted laughter. | Client does not seem interested in client, or vice versa; Interview seems dry and dull; Client and/or applicant seems uncomfortable; Interview does not last very long. |

## Caregiver nurtured by client:

| Green Lights | Red Flags |
| --- | --- |
| Client seems to enjoy conversing with applicant; Applicant behaves maturely, and not like an adored child with client. | Applicant talks over others in the room who are speaking to the client (attention stealing); Applicant being flirty with client; Applicant being overly dramatic about how difficult life is for him or her; Applicant going overboard to impress. |

## Caregiver controlled by client:

| Green Lights | Red Flags |
|---|---|
| Applicant seems comfortable and makes at least average eye contact with client; Applicant has questions when asked; Applicant appears at least moderately confident when answering client's questions; Applicant appears secure. | Applicant has difficulty making eye contact with client, and frequently looks down or away when speaking; Applicant overly nervous; Applicant sits with legs and or arms crossed, possibly rhythmically bouncing foot; Client talks down to applicant; Client insults client, even jokingly; Client rolls eyes at client during interview. |

## Caregiver who controls client:

| Green Lights | Red Flags |
|---|---|
| Applicant is polite to applicant, allows applicant to speak without interruption; Applicant responds to client, rather than the other way around; Applicant does not answer a question with a question; Client maintains a good eye contact with applicant; Client not agitated during interview; Applicant refers to client as "Sweetie." | Client seems tense; Applicant takes control of the interview; Applicant's eye contact with client is not reciprocated; Applicant stands over applicant, rather than sitting with client; Applicant places hands on hips; Applicant talks over client, or client does not talk at all. Applicant not overly confident or overbearing. |

The green lights and red flags are not an end all determination of a suitable fit, as some great caregivers are lousy at interviews, while some bad caregivers are highly skilled at acing them. When a hiring error is made, it can undone. If an applicant does poorly on only one of the tests, it does not have to be a deal breaker; however if the applicant seems to do badly on nearly every item, it might turn out to be a miserable match. First and foremost, rate the applicant on how well he or she does with *client* interaction – not the interaction with you – as the element relationship with you will likely be very different than with the client.

Janet Ng

# On the Job

*"Our society must make it right and possible for old people not to fear the young or be deserted by them, for the test of a civilization is the way that it cares for its helpless members."* –Pearl S. Buck

Good caregivers work hard. I personally believe the "great ones" who have worked with my mother deserve medals, as she is not an easy client. She has numerous health issues, needs assistance to transfer, and is frequently unkind due to cognitive decline. I have watched caregivers suffer ridicule and harassment, while being hit, scratched, spit on, and pinched – and continue to show up day after day. I have also seen caregivers walk out after 90 seconds. I totally understand why some  choose not to be there, but some return over and over. Perhaps the ones who return day after day are the truly experienced ones who understand cognitive decline, take it in stride, and fulfill their obligation to be good caregivers – or *more than likely they were born of an element compatible with the client.* The ones who walk out nearly always  have elements that contrast my mother's wood element. I have learned to ask every caregiver who walks through the door what her birthdate is to predict what is about to transpire between she and my mother.

Caregivers sent from an agency come without a personal interview with Mom – usually whomever they have willing to work with Mom; so the value of the interview is missing, and must be studied completely on the job, which is not altogether bad as we get to try them out before hiring privately; yet Mom has had to put up with emotional upset from a parade of failed care relationships before finding "the right one," when using the agency. On the other hand, interviewing for private caregivers from the Internet has not been a total success as people do not always behave on the job as in the interview.

The perfect middle occurs when the agency sees the merit of element compatibility, which lessens their turnover grief, as well. We have a good relationship with the agency, and they allow us to buy out a caregiver contracts for a fraction of the customary fee when they send a good match to my mother's door.

Once a caregiver is on the job, via private interview or agency-sent, the task of watching closely is critical. The green lights and red flags from the interview chapter can also be used as signs of ongoing compatibility. *Make it easy*. Install cameras with both video and audio. Let all caregivers know about the cameras. The idea is not to *catch* anyone behaving badly, but to *deter* mistreatment, and *study* the relationships. I have seen it all with my mother's cameras – even her mistreatment of the caregivers. The cameras not only protect the client, but also the caregiver.

There surely are evil caregivers who do mistreat vulnerable clients behind closed doors, leaving the client's cry for help sometimes ignored when family members are told that Mom was just confused. The same can occur the other way around where the client mistreats the caregiver, or tells an awful story about him or her that came from mixing dream with reality.

With the use of video/audio cameras that constantly record, you can easily get at the truth – which can also help with coaching. For example, there is a specific, non-standard method used to transfer Mom from her chair. When the technique is used, the transfer goes smoothly with no strain on the caregiver or Mom. When not done correctly, it can lead to injury to one or both. After the last time Mom fell from a maverick transfer, I decided to comb through video footage to find an excellent transfer. A 20-second video clip now goes to the phone of every caregiver who cares for my mother, and she has not fallen since. Cameras are equally nice for watching interactions for training purposes.

Review videos often, as well as watching live. It is here you will find great caregivers, as well as weed out bad matches.

Be especially alert if a caregiver with a controlling element is on duty. He or she may eventually forget or cease to care about the cameras, and show some unexpected, inappropriate behavior. I very rarely need to watch intently when a compatible caregiver is with Mom, as the relationship eventually becomes predictable, allowing me to relax. I always watch new caregivers closely, regardless the element, but after a while feel safe to turn the camera off if things are going well. If something does goes wrong, and I get a call from my mother or her caregiver, I am able to review footage via my phone, tablet, or computer. Without the cameras, I would miss out on so many good and not-so-good happenings. The camera has essentially become my mother's lifeline to me, as well as the caregivers' witness.

Do reward excellent care with tips, bonuses, time off, or some other perk to let the caregiver know the depth of your appreciation. Listen to the caregivers, as well as the client when bad interactions happen. There are two sides to every story. Do not disregard a client's version just because he or she has dementia, or otherwise cognitively challenged. I have found some of my mother's most bizarre-sounding stories to be mostly true, after reviewing video footage.

Do try to coach a failing caregiver before terminating – unless the offense was clearly abuse or neglect – as caregivers are often willing to listen and change something that is unacceptable to the client's care. Do pay attention to the relationship between the caregiver's and your elements so you can maximize compatibility in your supervisory role. Do establish boundaries between yourself and the caregiver to avoid being steam-rolled, or otherwise pushed around by a caregiver's desire to be unaccountable for his or actions and responsibilities. Do give second chances to failing caregivers where you see potential for change. Do stay involved with every aspect of care, as caregivers make mistakes, just like anyone else. Your involvement can help remedy situations that may lead to an accident. Most of all, reward excellent care, coach subpar care, and terminate abusive or neglectful care.

Janet Ng

# Tribute to My Mother

I would like to pay a special tribute to my mother who is mentioned so many times in this book, sometimes in a less than positive light. My mother has suffered from cognitive decline over the past few years, which has affected her personality and moods in a negative manner, causing frequent agitation, irritability, depression, and anger toward others – making her difficult to be around, at times.

This book does not refer to the woman she was before her decline, so I would like to do that now. Although this book is not about her, but rather about using Feng shui elements to choose compatible caregivers. She is nonetheless mentioned often as a vantage point for examples related to this book's focus. Yet because her behavior is frequently mentioned by example throughout this book, I would like to give her honor for the woman she was most of her life.

I can tell you from a front row seat that she was a spectacular mother, always making sure I had everything I needed. My family did not have an abundance, but we had enough, and I felt well cared for. She, with my father, raised me, along with my siblings, with more love, kindness, and respect than many other children receive growing up.

My mother went to work once all her children were in school, holding responsible positions throughout her career, and well-liked among the business community. She served as the executive director at a local chamber of commerce, which is the only job she still recalls today; but she also directed day care businesses, even designed with blueprint a day care building, for which she received special recognition. She was adored by children and parents, alike.

She sang professionally, and won best actress award within the local civic theatre for her role as Vita Louise in the play, "Harvey." To this day, she can belt out "Amazing Grace" like nobody's business.

My mother is a highly intelligent woman, and to this day can outthink her caregivers, and maintains an impeccable vocabulary. She has always been a decent woman, kind, helpful to others, and got along well with those she knew and worked with. She was generous to a fault, deeply caring for other's needs. Her late husband, whom she married many years after my father's death, developed dementia. She suffered the stress of caring for him, alone, before she, herself, began to suffer a different type of cognitive decline. Perhaps the stress of caring for him brought on her decline, or perhaps she was predisposed for it. Yet looking back, I saw where she frequently put her own needs aside to take care of him, and literature shows that stress can be a factor leading to cognitive issues.

My mother was a good woman, a kind woman, always putting others ahead of herself. It is difficult to frequently see the very opposite in her now, although at times her former self manages presence, and those are the moments I find joy in.

She is pictured on the front cover of this book as a child, dancing happy and free. This kind of existence is what I have tried to provide her at this time in her life by finding the best caregivers possible to bring light into her otherwise dismal days.

Thank you for reading my book, and I hope you found it helpful for your loved one, your clients, or yourself.


--Janet Ng

Janet Ng

# About the Author

Janet Ng holds a master's degree in Social Psychology from Ball State University. She worked in the addictions field, counseling and designing programs for over ten years in Indiana and Houston, Texas. She currently lives and works in San Antonio, Texas as a senior reporting analyst for a large healthcare company.

Janet created and maintained a website for several years, "Feng Shui Made Easy!" which received awards from other Feng shui sites, including Lillian Too's "World of Feng Shui". Janet provided personal reports to website visitors regarding home and office arrangement based on Feng shui, blended with relationship pointers based on elements. She received excellent feedback from many repeat customers who followed her tips.

Janet has managed her elderly mother's home care for the past few years, which has included hiring and coaching caregivers. A high turnover rate motivated her to put her social psychology degree, counseling experience, and Feng shui expertise to work to find more compatible and lasting companions to care for her mother.

www.ingramcontent.com/pod-product-compliance
Lightning Source LLC
Chambersburg PA
CBHW061439180526
45170CB00004B/1478